"Previously, the skin wa barrier. Now, we know t chemicals put on it, evel

This is an excellent overview of safe cosmetics and ... es to use on the skin. Dr. Farlow gives knowledgeable practical advice to people who want to have optimal health and makes it easy to choose safe and healthy products."

Peter Eckhart, M.D.
Women's Therapeutic Institute

"This book is a must read for people concerned with their health and those who have not been able to find the cause of some of their nagging health problems.

In this well researched and well presented book we learn of some of the limitations of the Food and Drug Administration in protecting our health. We also learn the truth about the chemicals used in cosmetics and personal care products that we use on a daily basis – products that may be contributing to the epidemic of obesity and the rapid rise in the incidence of such medical conditions as diabetes, asthma, irritable bowel syndrome, seizures, heart irregularities, migraine headaches, and neurological diseases."

Jack L. Samuels
President
Truth in Labeling Campaign

"What a gift! Buy this book for everyone you love. More and more we're learning to take care of ourselves from the inside out. Now Dr. Farlow has done the research and organized the information we need to be wise consumers and take care of our health from the outside in too. She has given us a simple, convenient and user-friendly tool to make responsible choices in our cosmetic and personal care purchases. This little book is a compact reference guide to take shopping with easy to locate ingredient list, ratings, safety tips, safe products, and complete resource information. Well done! We may live in a toxic world but we can change that! Thank you, Dr. Farlow for your knowledgeable guidance."

Connie Adams, CMT, FCCI
Certified Aromatherapy Instructor

"This book is an indispensable guide that translates the chemical 'gobbledy-gook' on product labels into understandable language. It makes it easy to confidently choose safe and healthy products. The writing style is easy reading and there are extensive verifiable references. No one should be without its wisdom. Thank you for making it possible."

Robert "Bob" Chew
Co-founder, A Better Community For All

"A must-read for time-starved parents! This book takes very complex material and distills it down to information that is credible and very quick and easy to read. Choosing healthy personal care products becomes easy because Dr. Farlow has done the hard work for you."

John Kjenner, CPA

"Thank you for such an informative book. I'm concerned about the ingredients in my health care products, and really appreciate the fact the ingredients can be found in one concise book. I've used the book to review ingredients in products I had been using and will be changing them because of the more informed decisions I'm able to make because of the information in this book."

Cheryl Strong

"I don't claim to know it all, by any means, but even from the little I know, your work must be done; it must be passed on to those of us who want to be enlightened so that we may use, first, safe and then beneficial personal use products.

Best wishes and congratulations on picking an important topic few would even know where to start to mine the gems you have already found."

German Ruiz
The Vital Image

"Great title and a great handbook to use when determining how healthy the products I use on myself and my animals really are. After reading the first few chapters, I wanted to make a trip to the store and read the ingredients listed for the products I use. Christine has also included a section of products that are safe, and provided an easy way to order them. There is no reason to continue to use unhealthy products!"

Martha Webb

"Dr. Farlow's work brings us the knowledge that it's not only what we put inside our bodies that affects our health, but what we put on the outside of our bodies affects our health too. The skin is an organ of the body that absorbs both nutrients and toxins. The fewer toxins we repeatedly put on our skin, the less risk we have at developing serious illnesses, like cancer. I highly recommend this guide book to all those who want to know how to take better care of themselves."

Joshua Leibow.
BA in Psychobiological Medicine
UC Santa Cruz

"This work is a good reference for most of us who don't have time to read all the latest information on ingredients and additives. Making it part of a regular routine to make healthy product choices can only improve one's physical health."

Chuck 'n Leslee Gervais

"Maybe we should call this book The Cosmetic Product Guide and the Natural Personal Care Product Bible. I was shocked at what some of the ingredients in my shampoo, deodorant, toothpaste, and sunscreen can do to my health. Now, I've got a list of safe and healthy personal care products. Do your health a favor; read and use this book."
- Larry Gibbs
Paralegal, researcher

"Some people will do anything to look good in their coffins. ... Every person who uses cosmetics – male or female – should have this book when they go shopping, or look up the products they are currently using."
Lendon H. Smith, M.D.
Author of *How to Raise a Healthy Child*

"Loved your little book. It is very informative, and gets to the real data pronto. Anyone who uses these chemicals on a daily basis would do well to get a copy of your book and read it. It is also wonderful as a reference."
Dr. Bruce West
Health Alert

"For years, I avoided cosmetics because of the fragrances or smothering effects I experienced when using them. ... Everyone concerned with looking good and being healthy needs this book to learn how to shop for cosmetics and health care products."
Ann P. Tidwell, Ph.D.
1st EnviroSafety

"This handy book slips into my purse so nicely, I will never again shop for cosmetics or toiletries without it. Once again I am reminded that personal responsibility is the key to personal well being. Your book makes this job easier."
Barbara Van Horne, DC

"We've been looking for a "non-biased" book on personal care products that's easy to follow and would allow us to assess products on our own by their ingredients. Your book is exactly what we were hoping to find."

Lisa Giordano, CNHP & Gregory Giordano, RN, CMT

"Your book is a truly useful reference guide. I've been checking labels since reading it and referencing back to your book. I never thought commercial toothpaste was particularly healthy, I just never realized before that it was a potentially deadly poison. It's in the wastebasket as is the can of shaving cream. And more, I'm sure, is yet to follow."

Bryan Stern, L.Ac.

"Finally! A compact, incredibly useful book that demystifies the labels on cosmetics. I have always hated the idea of putting toxic substances on my face--especially on my mouth and eyes--but labels never really helped me be a cautious consumer because the ingredients read like a foreign language. This book is a very valuable tool that I carry with me whenever I go shopping. Knowledge is power when it comes to fighting the battle against toxins. I love it!"

Stephanie Davis

Dying To Look Good:

The Disturbing Truth About What's Really in Your Cosmetics, Toiletries and Personal Care Products ...

And What You Can Do About It

Christine Hoza Farlow, D.C.

Second Edition, Completely Revised

KISS For Health Publishing
"Keep It Simple Secrets For Health"

DYING TO LOOK GOOD

The Disturbing Truth About What's Really In Your Cosmetics, Toiletries And Personal Care Products... And What You Can Do About It

Published by:

KISS For Health Publishing
P.O. Box 462335
Escondido, CA 92046-2335

Copyright © 2001, 2006 by Christine Hoza Farlow, D.C.
First Edition 2001
Second Edition 2006, completely revised

Printed in the United States of America

ISBN 0-9635635-6-4

Every effort has been made to insure the accuracy of the information in this book. However, nothing in this book should be construed as medical advice or used in place of medical consultation.

Acknowledgements

In doing the research for this book and updating the information from the previous edition, I have attempted to be as accurate as possible. This has not been an easy task. I have many people to thank for their assistance and input who made my job much easier than it might otherwise have been.

I thank Tanya Workman of Terra Naturals for sharing with me an outstanding series of well researched current articles on the many aspects of risks associated with the use of cosmetics and personal care products.

I thank Diana Kaye of Terressentials for sharing her knowledge and expertise from research she has done over the years in developing her own pure and natural product line and for offering her feedback on what I have written.

I thank Jack Samuels of the Truth in Labeling Campaign for making sure the information I present on MSG in Cosmetics is accurate. I also appreciate his great attention to detail and his valuable editorial assistance.

I thank Connie Adams for contributing her expertise in essential oils. Her depth of understanding in essential oils and their chemistry was truly helpful in rating the safety of essential oils as ingredients in cosmetics and personal care products.

I thank Lori Stryker of The Organic Makeup Company for sharing her expertise in the area of micronized minerals and the use of titanium dioxide and zinc oxide in cosmetics. I also appreciate her delightfully fresh and open way of thinking during our e-mail exchanges.

I thank Peter Eckhart, M.D. for sharing his expertise in the area of xenoestrogens, an area where he has devoted a considerable amount of research, and pointing me toward valuable resources in other areas as well.

I am very appreciative of the Environmental Working Group and their permission to use whatever I want of their information as long as I credit them properly. The work and research that went into producing the "Skin Deep" report on their website produced much needed facts and data that is not available anywhere else. Being able to access it for this book saved me a tremendous amount of time in my own research.

I thank my coach, Maria Marsala, who kept me focused and on track, and helped me to keep things in perspective.

I thank my daughter, Melissa, for being patient and understanding while I've spent so much time working on this book.

Last, but not least, I thank everyone who has offered any comments or suggestions that I have not mentioned here. Every comment, whether implemented or not, has been taken to heart and has contributed to the final outcome of this book.

Contents

HOW TO USE THIS BOOK

The codes below are to the left of each additive and indicate the safety of the additive when used for intended purposes in cosmetics and toiletries.

* *   GRAS - Generally Recognized As Safe by the FDA.

φ   FDA approved colorant

†   CIR (Cosmetic Ingredient Review) Expert Panel considers this ingredient safe

S   There is no known toxicity. The additive appears to be safe.

A   The additive may cause allergic reactions.

C   Caution is advised. The additive may be unsafe, poorly tested, or used in too many products we use on a regular basis.

C1   Caution is advised for certain groups in the population, such as pregnant women, infants, persons with high blood pressure, kidney problems, etc.

X   The additive is unsafe or very poorly tested.

For for quick and easy reference, print a copy of these codes from www.dyingtolookgood.com

Why You Should Use This Book

Your health is affected not only by what you put *into* your body in terms of food, drink, drugs and nutritional supplements, but also by what you put *on* your body. Your skin is not an impenetrable barrier as was thought years ago. We now know that all chemicals that come in contact with the skin can penetrate the skin in varying degrees. Many of the chemicals that can be absorbed through the skin have been detected in the blood stream.

Many of the ingredients used in cosmetics and personal care products are toxic, even though they may not cause any reactions on the skin. Some cause cancer. Some of the most commonly used ingredients combine with other ingredients to form cancer-causing substances.

In 2004, the Environmental Working Group evaluated the ingredients in 7,500 personal care products for safety. They found that:

- "One of every 120 products on the market contains ingredients certified by government authorities as *known or probable human carcinogens*, including shampoos, lotions, make-up foundations, and lip balms."
- "Seventy-one hair dye products contain ingredients derived from carcinogenic coal tar."
- "Fifty-five percent of all products assessed contain 'penetration enhancers,' ingredients that can increase a product's penetration through the skin and into the bloodstream, increasing consumers' exposures to other ingredients as well." Fifty of these products also contained "penetration enhancers in combination with known or probable human carcinogens."
- "Nearly 70 percent of all products contain ingredients that can be contaminated with impurities linked to cancer and other health problems."

- "Fifty-four products violate recommendations for safe use set by the industry's self-regulating Cosmetic Ingredient Review (CIR) board."
- And nearly all the products (99.6%) "contain one or more ingredients never assessed for potential health impacts by the CIR."

The cosmetics industry is very poorly regulated. The Federal Food, Drug, and Cosmetic (FD&C) Act does not require cosmetics and personal care products or their ingredients to be approved before they are marketed and sold to consumers. FDA regulation starts *after* they are already in the marketplace. So, except for color additives and a few ingredients, which are banned, manufacturers may use whatever ingredients they choose in the cosmetics and personal care products they produce without approval from the FDA.

However, the Fair Packaging and Labeling Act requires cosmetic manufacturers to list the ingredients on the label of every cosmetic and personal care product sold directly to consumers in descending order of quantity. In other words, the ingredient present in the largest quantity appears first on the label and the ingredient present is the smallest quantity appears last.

Cosmetic and personal care product manufacturers are not required to prove the claims they make about their products or to test their products for safety. However, if the product's safety has not been established, the product requires the label to state: "WARNING: The safety of this product has not been determined." According to EWG in their evaluation, they did not find a single product with this warning on the label.

Hair coloring products are among the most poorly regulated consumer products. There is no requirement to place a warning on the label of hair coloring products to inform consumers that these products cause cancer. Although the industry maintains that hair dyes are safe, there is a growing body of scientific evidence pointing to an increased risk of bladder cancer and non-Hodgkin's lymphoma associated with the use of permanent hair dyes.

According to John Bailey, Ph.D., director of the FDA'S Office of Cosmetics and Colors, "Consumers believe that 'if it's on the market, it can't hurt me,' and this belief is sometimes wrong."

The FDA can make suggestions or recommendations to manufacturers about cosmetic products or their ingredients, but *the manufacturers do not have to comply*. The FDA must first prove in a court of law that a product is harmful, improperly labeled, or violates the law if it wants to remove a cosmetic product from the market.

According to EWG, "The regulatory vacuum in the U.S. gives cosmetic companies tremendous leeway in selecting ingredients, while it transfers potentially significant and largely unnecessary health risks to the users of the products."

The requirement to list cosmetic and personal care product ingredients on the label applies to retail products sold for home use. Products produced for use in salons, labeled "For Professional Use Only" and cosmetic and personal care product samples do not require the ingredients to be listed on the label. However, these products do require the name of the distributor, the quantity, and all necessary warning statements.

Cosmetic, Toiletry and Fragrance Association

The Cosmetic, Toiletry and Fragrance Association (CTFA) is an industry organization supporting creative freedom in product development and self-regulation within the personal care product sector. It is the industry lobby at the various government levels.

The CTFA International Buyers' Guide 2004 edition lists over 12,000 cosmetic chemicals according to INCI names cross-referencing them to more than 55,000 trade and technical names.

INCI, International Nomenclature Cosmetic Ingredient, standardizes the terminology for cosmetic chemical ingredients in the U.S., Europe, Japan and other countries throughout the world. Manufacturers use this guide to choose their ingredients for the cosmetics they produce. Most of the chemicals have not been tested for short-term or long-term toxic effects or for systemic effects. Many are contaminated with toxic by-products from manufacturing. Many are toxic themselves.

The Cosmetic Ingredient Review

The Cosmetic Ingredient Review (CIR), established in 1976 by CTFA, was the industry's effort to provide an unbiased evaluation of the safety of cosmetic ingredients. Between 1976 and June 14, 2005, they completed safety assessments, for 1269 ingredients. This represents only 10% of the more than 12,000 ingredients listed in the International Cosmetic Ingredient Dictionary.

New cosmetic ingredients are coming onto the market faster than they can be reviewed. The 2004 edition of the International Cosmetic Ingredient Dictionary listed over 1400 more ingredients than were listed in the 2002 edition. In just two years more ingredients were added to the International Cosmetic Ingredient Dictionary than the CIR has reviewed in 29 years.

The CIR website states that they determine which ingredients to review based upon how widespread the use of the ingredient is and reports of adverse effects, toxicity predictions, potential for skin penetration, if banned in Japan or the European Union, etc. However, according to the

Environmental Working Group, based upon their review of the ingredients in 7,500 products in 2004, "the CIR has failed to review one-third of the top 50 ingredients used in cosmetics," some of which pose "potential cancer risks." In addition, "of the 1175 ingredients that had been reviewed by the CIR at the time of EWG's analysis, half of the ingredients are not used in cosmetics."

The EWG further states that "for many of the ingredients the CIR has chosen to review, the cosmetic industry has failed to conduct even the most basic toxicity tests."… For more than half of the ingredients approved by the CIR, "the panel fails in whole to discuss any available data with respect to cancer and mutagenicity, birth defects, and other reproductive risks." … The "CIR has chosen sensitization and the related effect of irritation as the basis for approximately 80% of its safety decisions, to the near total exclusion of other health impacts. … It is clear from the review summaries published by the panel in the open scientific literature that basic safety data are often lacking."

The CIR is funded by CTFA.

Buyer Beware

The FDA's attempt at establishing official definitions for specific terms like "natural" and "hypoallergenic" were overturned in court. Consequently, companies can use these terms on cosmetic labels to mean anything they want. Mostly, the value of these terms lies in promoting cosmetic products to the consumer rather than any real medical meaning, according to dermatologists.

Beware of products claiming to be:

- **Natural** – suggests that the ingredients are *derived* from natural sources rather than being produced synthetically. However, *there are no industry standards for what*

natural means. The product may contain all natural ingredients, just a few natural ingredients added to a synthetic product or even no natural ingredients at all.

- **Hypoallergenic** – means that the manufacturer believes the product is *less likely* to cause allergic reactions. But there are no standards for classifying a product hypoallergenic. The manufacturer may actually test the product before classifying it hypoallergenic, or simply remove fragrances and call it hypoallergenic. ***The manufacturer is not required to prove this claim.*** Also, the terms "dermatologist-tested," "sensitivity tested," "allergy tested," or "nonirritating" do not guarantee they won't cause allergic reactions.

- **Alcohol Free** – generally means the product does not contain ethyl alcohol (or grain alcohol). The product may contain fatty alcohols like cetyl, cetearyl, stearyl, or lanolin.

- **Fragrance Free** – means that the product has no detectable odor. ***Fragrance ingredients may still be added*** to mask offensive odors from the materials used to make the product.

- **Noncomedogenic** – implies that there are no pore-clogging ingredients that may cause acne in the product.

- **Cruelty Free** – suggests that there has been no animal testing of the product. In reality, the majority of cosmetic ingredients have been tested on animals at some point. A more accurate statement would be "no new animal testing," if indeed this were the case.

- **Shelf Life** (Expiration Date) – gives the length of time a cosmetic product is good if handled and stored properly. Expiration dates are approximate, and in reality, ***a product may expire long before the expiration date***.

- **And other ingredients** – means that there are one or more ingredients that the manufacturer considers a trade secret and does not want to list on the label. According to the FDA, "the manufacturer must prove that the ingredient imparts some unique property to the product and that the ingredient is not well-known in the industry."

Safety Tips

Here are a few tips to help you use your cosmetics and personal care products safely and protect yourself from harm associated with their misuse.

- Never apply makeup while driving. An accidental scratch to your eyeball can cause bacterial infection and result in serious injury, including blindness.

- Never share makeup, and certain personal care products, like toothpaste and deodorant.

- Be wary of testers at cosmetic counters. The product may be contaminated. If you must test before purchasing, insist on a new disposable applicator and that the salesperson clean the container opening with alcohol before applying to your skin.

- Never add liquid to a cosmetic product to restore its original consistency. This may cause bacterial contamination.

- Stop using a product if you've had an allergic reaction to it.

- Throw away products in which there has been a change in color or odor.

- Do not use eye makeup if you have an eye infection. Discard all products you were using when you discovered the infection.

- Keep makeup out of sunlight.

- Close makeup containers tightly when not in use.

- Many aerosol products are flammable. Do not use near heat or while smoking. Do not inhale hairsprays and powders. They may cause lung damage.

Special Topics

There are some products on the market that people use, …
just because everyone does, or because they make your face,
skin, hands, hair or teeth look beautiful, or because the
manufacturer, through their million dollar advertising
campaigns has convinced you that you just can't live without
it. That it will make you more beautiful, sexier and will lure
your perfect partner to you.

Until recently, most people didn't even think about what's in
the product or if it's even safe to put on their skin. They just
thought about what it's going to do for them, how it's going
to make them look or feel and how attractive it will make
them to the opposite sex.

But that's changing now. There's a growing consciousness
toward using safer and healthier products. And it's turning
out that a number of the products that people just took for
granted because of what it "did for them," are actually
causing harm.

As of this writing, there is a proposed bill in California,
which if passed, would require manufacturers to notify the
state of any products they manufacture that contain
ingredients linked to cancer or birth defects. EWG identified
155 products that would be affected if the bill passes. It
passed the California Assembly's Health Committee on June
28, 2005 and was placed on the Suspense Calendar until after
August 15.

According to EWG, "California's bill also opens the door for
national reform of loose standards for personal care products
that essentially have industry lobbyists in control of
determining if the ingredients their companies use are safe."
If this bill passes, it could be the first step in seeing safer
cosmetics available to consumers.

You can follow the developments in this and other environmental safety issues at www.ewg.org.

Here's a brief look at some topics, that you should be aware of, that are important to your health, including both products and ingredients.

Acrylic Nails

Artificial nails, even though they may look great, are in fact harmful to your health and the health of your nails.

The chemicals used to attach and remove acrylic nails are toxic. Ethyl methacrylate most commonly used to glue on acrylic nails, is an eye and skin irritant. Inhaling it can cause headaches, dizziness and nausea. It can also cause asthma and allergic reactions.

Methyl methacrylate was banned in 1974 after it was proven harmful. It is still being used in some establishments "because it's cheap, effective and easy to get despite the ban," according to Evelyn Burgett, Cosmetology Inspector for the state of Tennessee.

Acrylic nails have been found to harbor bacteria, fungi and viruses. Significantly higher levels of these microorganisms have been detected on the hands of people with acrylic nails compared with those without.

Allergic reactions may occur when the chemicals come in contact with the skin surrounding the nails causing redness, swelling and itching to occur around the nail and even causing the nail to separate from the nail bed.

In addition, your nails are porous. Chemicals that come in contact with them can be absorbed through the nail bed into your bloodstream.

Antibacterial Soaps

Antibacterial soaps have been widely embraced as a way to "kill germs" and prevent illness. But not all bacteria are harmful. And not all "germs" are bacteria.

Some bacteria are beneficial and your body needs them. Antibacterial soaps cannot distinguish between harmful and helpful bacteria. It kills all bacteria. When the healthy bacteria that your body needs have been "washed away," it leaves you more susceptible to illness from harmful bacteria.

Recent studies show that triclosan, one of the most common antibacterial agents used in soaps, acts like an antibiotic in the way it kills bacteria and may contribute to the development of antibiotic resistant bacteria.

It has been suggested that antibacterial soaps should not be used on children because the chemicals are too harsh and drying for their skin. Using antibacterial soaps on your children does not protect them and help them to stay healthy. In fact, children need to come in contact with "germs" to help them to develop their immune system. Overuse of antibacterial agents has been linked to allergies and asthma.

And antibacterial agents do not kill viruses, the microorganisms responsible for colds and flu.

The Centers for Disease Control (CDC) says that the use of antibacterial soaps is not necessary on a daily basis. Washing with warm water and ordinary soap is sufficient.

Cosmetics Classified as Drugs

Cosmetic or personal care products that claim to have a therapeutic benefit affecting body function or structure are also classified as drugs.

These products often can be identified by an "active ingredient" listed in the label. But not all products in this category always list an active ingredient. They are only required to list the active ingredient first, then the remaining inactive ingredients.

The typical type of cosmetic products also considered drugs include:

- Fluoride toothpaste
- Dandruff shampoo
- Sunscreens
- Cosmetics containing sunscreen

Cosmetics That Require a Warning on the Label

The FDA requires warnings on the labels of products that are potentially hazardous, including:

- Aerosol products
  - Hairsprays
  - Deodorant
- Products in pressurized containers
  - Shaving cream
  - Foaming soaps
- Detergent bubble bath products
- Hair dyes containing coal tar colors
- Feminine deodorant sprays
- Shampoos, rinses and conditioners
- Hair straighteners and depilitories
- Nail builders (elongators, extenders, hardeners, and enamels)
- Any product that contains one or more ingredients that the CIR found had insufficient testing data to support the ingredients' safe use in cosmetics

According to the Environmmental Working Group, of the 7500 products they tested, nearly one in 20 contained one or more ingredients that the CIR found *did not* have sufficient test data to support the ingredients' safe use in cosmetics. Under federal law, passed in 1995, if a cosmetic product's safety has not been established, the product's label must read: "WARNING: The safety of this product has not been determined."

The EWG did not find any warnings on the labels of the products whose ingredients contained insufficient data to support safety, based on a partial evaluation. Unless studies were done to provide the information needed for these ingredients to be classified as safe, "the manufacturers of these products may be in violation of federal law."

In their evaluations, the EWG also noted that the industry routinely ignores the recommendations of the CIR on the safe use of ingredients as determined by the panel.

Grapefruit Seed Extract

The safety of grapefruit seed extract (GSE) is controversial. On the one hand, some companies are removing grapefruit seed extract from their products. On the other, some say it's non-toxic and has no harmful side-effects.

Grapefruit seed extract has been used for many years as a safe alternative to chemical preservatives. However, a study done in 1999 in Germany on six samples of grapefruit seed extract showed contamination with benzethonium chloride in five of the six samples tested. Three of these five samples were also found to contain triclosan and methyl paraben. Each of these samples showed antimicrobial activity. The one sample that contained no preservatives showed no antimicrobial activity. This study concluded that the antimicrobial activity of grapefruit seed extract was due to the chemical preservatives detected, not to the grapefruit seed extract.

Conversely, Nutribiotics, one of the major suppliers of grapefruit seed extract, states that their grapefruit seed extract products have been "proven clean" and effective by independent laboratory tests. They assert that grapefruit seed extract has been used safely for many years. It is "non-toxic, biodegradable, economical, with no harmful side-effects."

So, when choosing products containing grapefruit seed extract, make sure the grapefruit seed extract in the products you choose comes from a reputable source with independent lab tests to verify safety and effectiveness. Quality, safety and effectiveness of grapefruit seed extract may vary among different brands.

Hair Dyes*

The industry maintains that "hair dyes are one of the most thoroughly studied consumer products on the market today" and they're safe. However, there is a growing body of scientific evidence pointing to an increased risk of bladder cancer and non-Hodgkin's lymphoma associated with the use of permanent hair dyes, especially the darker colors.

Here are some facts about hair dyes reported in "Shades of Risk," by Shelley Page:

"A study published in the January/February 2005 issue of Public Health Reports, the official journal of the U.S. Public Health Service, found that the use of permanent hair dyes among men and women increases the risk of developing bladder cancer by up to 50 per cent compared to those who don't use hair dye."

In 2004, a "study by Yale researcher Tongzhang Zheng found that long-term use of permanent hair dye, in dark colors, doubles a person's risk of non-Hodgkin's lymphoma"

"The EU watchdog, known as the Scientific Committee on Cosmetic and Non-Food Products Intended for Consumers (SCCNFP), is worried about fatal allergies caused by hair dyes, as well as "new and improved" studies linking dyes to cancer. SCCNFP has strongly criticized hair-dye manufacturers for failing to prove hair dyes are safe and has ordered urgent research to be conducted on the health implications of permanent hair dyes or the product could face a ban. In the meantime, it has warned consumers not to use hair dyes, particularly dark dyes."

"Researchers from the University of Southern California's (USC) School of Medicine found in 2001 that women using permanent hair dye at least once a month more than double their risk of bladder cancer. If they used it monthly for more than 15 years, they tripled their risk. The risk of bladder cancer was highest among smokers who regularly used hair dyes."

In 2003 the FDA's National Center for Toxicological Research reported that it found a known carcinogen, 4-ABP, in eight of 11 hair dye products bought off the shelf at supermarkets and hair salons. It was not listed as a regular ingredient, but was likely a contaminant formed as a byproduct of the dye-making process according to the researchers.

In the summer of 2004, the Environmental Working Group (EWG) analyzed 117 hair dyes. It found:

- 62 per cent of products contained ingredients that are known or probable carcinogens, including dyes derived from coal tar
- One product contained lead acetate, a known reproductive toxin
- 79 per cent of products contained ingredients that contained impurities linked to breast cancer
- 96 per cent of products contained penetration enhancers that increase exposures to carcinogens and other ingredients of concern
- 73 per cent of products contained ingredients that are known allergens.

Here's the EWG's list of Top 10 Ingredients of Concern in Hair Dye based upon their research:

- P-phenylenediamine
- P-animophenol
- M-aminophenol
- Phenyl Methyl Pyrazolone
- 4-amino-2-hydroxytoluene
- 1-naphthol
- N-phenyl-p-phenylenediamine
- O-aminophe+nol
- Lead acetate
- HC Red No. 3

*Excerpted and modified from "Shades of Risk" by Shelley Page, published in the Ottawa Citizen, April 18, 2005. Used with permission.

Micronized Minerals

Micronized minerals are emerging on the marketplace in natural cosmetics and sunscreens. Many companies promoting natural cosmetics are extolling the benefits of micronized minerals in their "all natural" make-up. Some cosmetic products are promoted as 100% pure micronized minerals

But beware! There are research studies that suggest caution when considering the use of micronized mineral cosmetics.

Micronized minerals, also known as ultrafine or nanoparticles, are mineral pigments where the size of the particles has been reduced. In general, particles are classified according to size as coarse, fine or ultrafine. Micronized particles, the ultrafine or nanoparticles, are 100 times smaller than coarse particles and 25 times smaller than fine particles, according to etcgroup.org.

According to the FDA, there is no *official* definition of "micronized," but they refer to these particles being less than 250 nanometers, and they also regard nanoscale titanium dioxide as "micronized titanium dioxide."

Studies have shown that ultrafine particles can penetrate the skin, enter the cell and cause DNA damage. There is concern that this could possibly result in skin cancer. These studies have been done on titanium dioxide.

As of 2005, "The National Toxicology Program is developing a broad-based research program to address potential human health hazards associated with the manufacture and use of nanoscale materials," using existing testing methods and developing new methods to "adequately assess potential adverse human health effects."

Currently, the FDA's National Center for Toxicological Research and the National Toxicology Program's Center for Phototoxicology are conducting research "to examine the potential dermal toxicity of nanoscale materials." In this study they are investigating titanium dioxide and zinc oxide.

Based upon the studies being done and in development, it appears that not only are micronized minerals not well defined and not adequately tested, but also, the technology necessary to adequately test them for safety has not yet been completely developed.

MSG In Your Personal Care Products

MSG is short for monosodium glutamate, but it also applies to processed free glutamic acid (glutamic acid that has been freed from protein through a manufacturing process or fermentation). I'm sure you're aware of MSG in food, the effects it can cause and the controversy surrounding its safety. But did you know that MSG could also be hidden in your cosmetics and personal care products?

When you use products on your skin that contain MSG, it's absorbed directly into your bloodstream.

MSG is a neurotoxin, which means it crosses the blood-brain barrier and the placental barrier and excites nerve cells to death. Because it affects the brain directly, it can cause a wide variety of symptoms from asthma attacks, skin rashes, behavioral problems, depression and migraine headaches to epilepsy and Alzheimer's.

Even more frightening is that MSG is much more harmful to infants and children because, in some, their blood-brain barrier does not fully develop until as late as puberty. As a result, it's a lot easier for neurotoxins to cross the blood-brain barrier in infants and children and cause more serious reactions than in adults. Even a fully developed blood-brain barrier is considered by neuroscientists to be leaky at best.

MSG is hidden in many products, besides food, that you use every day, including:

- cosmetics and personal care products
  - soaps
  - shampoos
  - conditioners
  - cosmetics
- nutritional supplements
- medications
- vaccines

You can identify MSG in your personal care products by reading the label and looking for specific ingredients that are always or often sources of hidden MSG.

MSG is always in ingredients like
- hydrolyzed proteins
- amino acids
- yeast extract

- nayad (potent yeast extract)
- glutamic acid
- glutamates.

MSG may also be in or be the result of
- processed proteins
- enzymes
- carrageenan.

These are the most likely sources of MSG in your personal care products. For a complete list of ingredients containing MSG, see truthinlabeling.org/hiddensources.html.

For more information on hidden sources of MSG, see truthinlabeling.org/II.WhereIsMSG.html.

Permanent Makeup

Permanent makeup is the process of infusing natural, mineral pigments under the skin's surface. This micropigmentation, a kind of tattooing, is designed to last many years.

But the convenience has its risks. The pigments used can be toxic and cause adverse reactions. According to the FDA, there have been numerous reports of adverse reactions, associated with a considerable number of Premier ink shades.

The inks and pigments used in permanent makeup are classified as cosmetics and color additives, which are subject to FDA regulation. However, the FDA has not regulated their use and has left it up to local jurisdictions. The FDA is just starting to look into the safety issues.

The FDA has two lists of approved colors for cosmetic use,
- those subject to batch certification, which are the FD&C, D&C and Ext. D&C colors
- those exempt from batch certification

None of the approved colors are approved to be injected into the skin, as is done with permanent makeup.

Risks Associated with Permanent Makeup

- Infections
- Allergic reactions
- Keloids
- Granulomas
- Dissatisfaction
- Removal problems

Allergic reactions may show up years later in the form of a rash or immune system reaction.

Dissatisfaction is a major problem with permanent makeup. If you don't like the result, removing it can be difficult. If the person applying your permanent makeup makes a mistake, you can't wash it off; you're either stuck with it, or you have to go through a removal process. Removal often isn't perfect and can leave scars. Over time, permanent makeup can fade or bleed. As your body changes, the appearance of your permanent makeup may change as well.

Adverse effects associated with permanent makeup include:

- Peeling
- Cracking
- Blistering
- Swelling
- Granulomas
- Scarring
- Disfigurement

And, what are the long-term effects on your body of the pigments injected under your skin?

According to chemist John Bailey, Ph.D., Director of FDA's Colors and Cosmetics Program, "we can't vouch for the safety of permanent eyelining because *the procedure hasn't undergone any formal safety testing*."

You can report adverse reactions to permanent makeup and tattoos by contacting:

Cosmetics Adverse Reaction Monitoring (CARM) System
Office of Cosmetics and Colors
HFS-106
Center for Food Safety and Applied Nutrition
Food and Drug Administration
5100 Paint Branch Parkway
College Park, MD 20740-3835
 (202) 401-9725.

Sunscreens

In our society, most people don't question the need for sunscreens. It's just accepted as the standard healthy practice when you plan to be out in the sun.

But beware! What's generally accepted as true is not necessarily true!

Here are some facts to consider before lathering that sunscreen all over yourself and your children the next time you go out into the sun:

- Sunscreens will not safeguard you from melanoma, a potentially deadly type of skin cancer. They don't filter or block the harmful melanoma-causing UVA rays; they only reduce sunburn risk.
- Sunscreens offer some protection against easily treatable basal cell carcinoma.
- Your body needs the UVB rays from the sun to produce vitamin D. Sunscreens, as low as SPF 8, block the UVB rays responsible for vitamin D synthesis.

- Sunscreens are regulated by the FDA as over-the-counter drugs because they contain active ingredients, many of which are toxic.
- Both chemical suncreens and physical sunblocks have been shown to cause the formation of free radicals with exposure to sunlight. Excess free radicals are known to cause cancer.
- A Swiss study showed that five commonly used chemicals in sunscreens were xenoestrogens, endocrine disrupters, and they actually increased the growth of cancer cells. See "Xenoestrogens in Your Personal Care Products," page 39.
- Most, if not all, sunscreens include a hydrolyzed protein. All hydrolyzed proteins contain processed free glutamic acid (MSG).
- Research has shown that excess omega-6 fats in the diet actually contribute to the occurrence of cancer, including melanoma.

Here are some tips on how to enjoy the sun safely without the hazards of sunscreen:

- Start out with 10 minutes of exposure a day and gradually increase your sun time.
- Limit time in the sun to morning before 10 a.m. or afternoon after 2 p.m. when the sun is not at its hottest.
- Cover up when outdoors during the sun's hottest times and when you've already had your quota of sun for the day.
- Avoid getting sunburned.

Eat a healthy balance of omega 3 and omega 6 fats. Most people eat far too much omega 6's and not enough omega 3's. Research has shown omega's 3's to be preventive against melanoma if eaten in the proper one-to-one balance with omega 6's. Omega 3 fats can be found in fish oils and flaxseed. You also need healthy saturated fats, like real butter or coconut oil, to utilize omega 3's.

"The Truth About Sunscreens," on the Terressentials web site, states that "sunscreens give users a false sense of security in that while they effectively prevent sunburn, they do little or nothing to prevent skin cancer or the accelerated aging of the skin caused by sunlight."

It further states that "There is a substantial body of evidence that shows that there is an increase in cancer when sunscreen products are used. We've done a lot of research into sunscreens. The bottom line is this: we have found no sunscreen ingredients which we consider to be safe."

Titanium Dioxide and Zinc Oxide Safety

Titanium dioxide and zinc oxide are typically used in sunscreen products and cosmetics and have been generally considered safe.

However, studies show that cellular damage from titanium dioxide, occurs with exposure to sunlight, and depends upon the type of titanium dioxide and the size of the particles. Cellular damage has been shown to occur when the particle size is smaller than the size of the cell. The smallest particles, the micronized or nanoparticles, are the most injurious. Some say that the large particles are less harmful, yet others say they're safe.

According to Lori Stryker of the Organic Makeup Company, who has done considerable research into the safety of titanium dioxide in its various forms, "if the particle size is too large for the cell membrane to allow it passage internally, then the danger of intracellular mutation is not there." Still, there are those who say that even the larger particles can pass through the skin to some degree, and are just less absorbable than the small particles. They suggest that even the larger particles may contribute some harm.

Obviously, the safety of the larger particles of titanium dioxide and zinc oxide is not well established and agreed upon within the scientific community. There is clearly a need for more research into the mechanism of how the larger sized particles of titanium dioxide and zinc oxide affect the skin and the cells beneath the skin when exposed to the sun.

Cautions regarding micronized titanium dioxide and zinc oxide, are discussed on page 31.

Xenoestrogens in Your Personal Care Products

Xenoestrogens are endocrine disrupters. They are chemicals that mimic estrogen in your body and interfere with the normal functioning of your hormones.

Endocrine disrupters are found in a great many personal care products on the market, including shampoos, conditioners, lotions, sunscreens, and cosmetics as well as baby products.

Estrogen mimicking chemicals have been implicated in early puberty in girls, development of breast cancer, some association with vaginal and cervical cancer, and endometriosis. In males, they have been associated with reproductive disorders, including decreased sperm count, increase in testicular cancer, hypospadias and cryptorchidism, and possibly benign prostatic hypertrophy and prostate cancer.

Women exposed to xenoestrogens during pregnancy may have children with reproductive disorders, sometimes not apparent till puberty. This exposure may also adversely affect the children's intelligence and behavior, as well as their immune system.

The xenoestrogens most commonly found in personal care products are the parabens:

- butylparaben
- ethylparaben

- methylparaben
- proplyparaben

Other xenoestrogens, used mostly in sunscreens, facial cosmetics and lipsticks include:

- octyl-methoxycinnamate
- octyl-dimethyl-PABA
- benzophenone-3
- homosalate
- 4-methyl-benzylidene camphor (4-MBC)

These five chemicals not only demonstrated strong estrogenic effects, but also caused increased growth of cancer cells in a Swiss study.

Most companies using parabens, maintain that they are nontoxic and safe. But while they may be relatively nontoxic, according to Peter Eckhart, M.D., "The new theory that has been espoused since 1991 is that these xenoestrogens are causing many female problems such as endometriosis, ovarian cysts, fibrocystic breast disease, premenstrual syndrome, and most recently menstrual cramps."

While it's true that xenoestrogens build up in the fatty tissues of the body and may remain there for decades, the first step in eliminating them from your body is through avoidance of the chemicals, not only in personal care products, but also in food and in your environment. The chemicals listed above are only a partial list of endocrine disrupters. The complete list and additional information can be obtained from www.womhoo.com.

Cosmetic complaints

The FDA maintains the Cosmetic Adverse Reaction
Monitoring Database to keep track of adverse reactions to
cosmetics. The FDA estimates, however, that it receives only
a small percentage of complaints about cosmetics filed by
consumers. Poison control centers, manufacturers and
distributors, and state and local agencies are more likely to
receive complaints of adverse reactions to cosmetics.

The most common complaints reported to the FDA in 1999
were related to dermatitis, fragrance sensitivity, nervous
system reactions, pain, respiratory system reactions, and
tissue damage.

If you experience adverse reactions to cosmetics, you can
contact the FDA:

- by phone: 301-436-2405
- by e-mail: CAERS@cfsan.fda.gov
- call the nearest FDA district office found in the blue
  pages of your phone book

How the Classifications Were Determined

Many references were used in determining how to classify each ingredient in this book according to safety. In addition to the references listed in the back of the book, available information was reviewed from the:

- Cosmetic Ingredient Review (CIR)
- Environmental Working Group (EWG)
- National Fire Protection Association (NFPA) Chemical Hazard Ratings
- National Toxicology Program (NTP) Report on Carcinogens
- International Agency for Research on Cancer (IARC)
- Material Safety Data Sheets (MSDS) from chemical manufacturers and various government agencies.

Not All Safety Ratings Agree With the FDA or CIR

In many cases, the various references were not in complete agreement as to the safety of the ingredient. In those cases, I have taken the conservative approach: if there is any indication from any of the sources that the ingredient might have any adverse effects, then they were noted and rated according to the significance or severity of the adverse reactions. In most cases, the references indicating the most severe reactions were given the most weight.

Oftentimes, in the "Cosmetic Ingredients" list, you will find ingredients that are GRAS (Generally Recognized As Safe), considered safe by the CIR or FDA approved colorants that are *not* rated **S** or safe. This is because, based upon all the information available to me, I did not agree with the CIR or FDA that these ingredients were in fact safe.

Ingredients are rated **X** if:
- they are known carcinogens, as determined through research studies

- the International Agency for Research on Cancer (IARC) gives them a Group 1, 2A or 2B rating
- are known to be unsafe for various reasons
- there's no safety data

Ingredients are rated **C** if:
- they're not carcinogenic, but may form a carcinogen by reacting with another ingredient in the product
- they're not carcinogenic, but may be contaminated with a carcinogen in the production of the ingredient
- the International Agency for Research on Cancer (IARC) gives them a Group 3 rating
- they may cause a variety of mild to moderate adverse effects
- they're considered safe, but there's inadequate safety data available

Ingredients are rated **C1** if:
- they may be harmful for certain groups of the population, i.e., children or pregnant women.

Ingredients are rated **S** if:
- they're known to be safe, supported by safety data
- known safe for the general population, but some people may have a mild reaction to the ingredient.

The safest products are products with the fewest number of ingredients and with the ingredients rated S. However, even if all of the ingredients used in our cosmetics and personal care products are safe individually, rarely does any product have only one ingredient in it. Safety testing has only been done for individual ingredients, not for combinations of ingredients. Ingredients safe individually may be harmful in certain combinations. ***Nobody knows the effects of the many different ingredients used in the thousands of different combinations, the effects of using numerous different products, one on top of the other, or the effects of repeated use of ingredients or products over time.***

IARC Classifications Regarding Cancer-Causing Risk

The International Agency for Research on Cancer evaluates data from scientific studies to determine whether there is a risk that the chemicals or mixtures are carcinogenic and classifies them into the following categories:

Group 1 – human carcinogen
Group 2A – probable human carcinogen
Group 2B – possible human carcinogen
Group 3 – cannot be classified as a human carcinogen
Group 4 –probably not a human carcinogen

Ingredients listed in this book are classified as a carcinogen only if there is supportive evidence of its carcinogenic status from IARC, or other agencies that are qualified to determine carcinogenic status. The IARC Group classification is listed for individual ingredients in the Cosmetic Ingredient listing.

For more detailed information and explanations of the IARC Group classifications, see:

"Lists of IARC Evaluations,"
    www-cie.iarc.fr/monoeval/grlist.html

"Preamble to the IARC Monographs,"
    www-cie.iarc.fr/monoeval/preamble.html

"Evaluation," www-cie.iarc.fr/monoeval/eval.html

"IARC Monographs on the Evaluation of Carcinogenic Risks to Humans," www-cie.iarc.fr

Natural vs. Synthetic

There are no standard definitions within the cosmetic and personal care product industry for natural or synthetic. However, the National Organic Program (NOP) does have definitions that are accepted within the organic food industry.

Since many people are interested in knowing if the ingredients in their products are natural or synthetic, the NOP definitions were used to define the ingredients in the Cosmetic Ingredient List as natural or synthetic:

Nonsynthetic (natural)

"A substance that is derived from mineral, plant, or animal matter and *does not* undergo a synthetic process as defined in section 6502(21) of the Act (7 U.S.C. 6502(21)). For the purposes of this part, nonsynthetic is used as a synonym for natural as the term is used in the Act."

Synthetic

"A substance that is formulated or manufactured by a chemical process or by a process that chemically changes a substance extracted from naturally occurring plant, animal, or mineral sources, except that such term shall not apply to substances created by naturally occurring biological processes."

Cosmetic and Personal Care Product Ingredients

S   Abies alba – see fir oil.

S   Abies sibirica – see fir oil.

X   4-ABP – synthetic; carcinogenic contaminant in some hair dyes; IARC Group 1.

C   Acetic ether – synthetic solvent; see ethyl acetate.

XA   Acetone – synthetic solvent; petroleum derivative; eye, nose, throat and skin irritant; may cause light headedness, nausea, coma, nail splitting, peeling and brittleness; lung irritant if inhaled; narcotic in large amounts; neurotoxin; has caused liver, kidney, and nerve damage in lab animals; extremely toxic.

X   Acetophenetidide – see phenacetin.

X   Acetophenetidin – see phenacetin.

X   Acetyl ethyl tetramethyl tetralin – synthetic; toxic to nervous system, may cause hyperirritability; has caused brain, spinal cord and nervous system damage and death in lab animals; absorbs through the skin.

†CA   Acetylated lanolin – skin irritant; may cause acne; see lanolin.

C1   Achillea millefolium – see yarrow oil.

X   Acid Blue 9 – synthetic; coal tar dye; carcinogen.

C   Acrylates copolymer – synthetic; petroleum derivative; may contain carcinogenic contaminants; CIR says safe when formulated to avoid irritation.

S   Aesculus hippocastanum - herb, anti-inflammatory, for sensitive skin, capillary fragility.

X   AETT – synthetic; see acetyl ethyl tetramethyl tetralin.

C   Alcohol – may be synthetic petroleum derivative or from fermented carbohydrates; can cause systemic contact dermatitis, eczema; see ethyl alcohol.

C   Alcohol C12 – synthetic; see lauryl alcohol.

C   Alkaline persulphates – synthetic; has caused asthma in hairdressers; contains ammonium salts, see ammonia.

CA   Alkanoamides – synthetic; may cause formation of carcinogenic nitrosamines in products containing nitrogen compounds; cause contact dermatitis.

C   Alkoxylated alcohols – synthetic; may contain dangerous levels of toxins.

C   Alkoxylated amides – synthetic; may cause formation of carcinogenic nitrosamines in products containing nitrogen compounds; cause contact dermatitis.

C   Alkoxylated amines – synthetic; may contain dangerous levels of toxins; see amines.

C   Alkoxylated carboxylic acids – synthetic; may contain dangerous levels of toxins.

C   Alkyl ether sulfates – synthetic; may cause formation of carcinogenic nitrosamines in products containing nitrogen compounds; cause contact dermatitis; contains ammonium salts, see ammonia.

C   Alkyl sulfates – synthetic; may cause dermatitis, irritate skin; contains ammonium salts, see ammonia.

C   Allantoin – herb; healing properties; may irritate skin; may be from plant sources or synthetically derived from uric acid; avoid synthetic sources; not believed to be a hazard; no toxicology data available; on CIR high priority review list.

C   Allantoin polygalacturonic acid group – see allantoin, galacturonic acid.

S   Allium sativum – herb, see garlic.

CA   Almond glycerides – synthetic; potential skin irritant; safety data not available.

SA   Almond oil – carrier oil; healing for irritated or dry skin; may irritate skin.

†S   Aloe – plant derived; herb, healing properties; antibacterial; anti-inflammatory; moisturizer; may be irrant for some; CIR says safe as used if anthraquinone levels in the ingredients do not exceed 50 ppm.

†S   Aloe extract – see aloe, extract.

†S   Aloe vera – see aloe.

S   Aloe vera gel – see aloe.

†S   Aloe vera juice – see aloe.

†S   Alpha-bisabolol – essential oil; component of chamomile; non-allergenic; anti-inflammatory; CIR says safe as used.

†C   Alpha hydroxy acids – synthetic combined with natural extracts; cause photosensitivity which subsides within a week of discontinuing use; has caused severe redness, blistering, burning, swelling, skin discoloration, itching, rashes; penetrates skin more deeply in cream base; oral administration in lab animals has caused kidney stones and nephrotoxic effects; safety of long-term use unknown; CIR panel says safe if concentration is 10% or less, pH is 3.5 or greater, and product is formulated so it protects the skin from increased sun sensitivity or tells consumer to use sun protection; or concentration is 30% or less, pH is 3 or greater in products designed for brief, discontinuous use , followed by a thorough rinsing from the skin, when applied by trained professionals, and when given directions for daily use of sun protection; European Union allows a maximum concentration of only 4%; not recommended for children.

†C   Alpha hydroxy and botanical complex – see alpha hydroxy acids.

†C   Alpha-hydroxycaprylic acid – see alpha hydroxy acids.

†C   Alpha-hydroxyethanoic acid + ammonium alpha-hydroxyethanoate – synthetic; see alpha hydroxy acids.

†C   Alpha-hydroxyoctanoic acid – synthetic; see alpha hydroxy acids.

C   Alpha-hydroxytoluene – synthetic; may cause contact dermatitis.

C   Alpha-methylquinoline – synthetic; skin irritant; see quinaldine.

C   Alpha-pinene – natural plant derivative; irritates skin, may cause contact dermatitis.

S   Althea extract – see marshmallow, extract.

S   Althea officinalis – see marshmallow.

CA   Aluminum chloride – synthetic; skin irritant; moderately toxic if swallowed.

CA   Aluminum chlorohydrate – synthetic; skin irritant; may cause hair follicle infections.

CA   Aluminum phenolsulfate – synthetic; skin irritant; contains ammonium salts, see ammonia, aluminum sulfate.

*CA   Aluminum sulfate – synthetic; skin irritant; moderately toxic if swallowed; not shown to be safe; ammonium salt, see ammonia.

φC   Aluminum powder – may be causative factor in Alzheimer's; inhalation can cause lung disease; see external use only.

C   Amines – synthetic; may cause formation of carcinogenic nitrosamines in products containing nitrogen compounds; cause contact dermatitis.

C   Amino acids – components of protein, some of which are necessary for health; includes glutamic acid, a non-essential amino acid; see MSG.

X   4-Aminobiphenyl – synthetic; see 4-ABP.

X   2-amino-4-nitrophenol – synthetic; skin irritant; may cause convulsions with skin contact; may cause asthma if inhaled; sensitizer; mutagen, may cause genetic damage; IARC Group 3.

X   2-amino-5-nitrophenol – synthetic; see 2-amino-4-nitrophenol.

†CA   4-amino-2-hydroxytoluene – synthetic; used in hair dyes; sensitizer, eye and skin irritant; CIR says safe as used.

X   4-amino-2-nitrophenol – synthetic; see 2-amino-4-nitrophenol.

X   4-aminobiphenyl – synthetic; carcinogenic contaminant in some hair dyes; IARC Group 1.

C   2-aminoethanol – synthetic; see ethanolamine.

†CA   Aminoform – synthetic; see methenamine.

†C   Aminomethyl propanol – synthetic; may irritate skin; used in concentrations up to 10%; not

adequately tested for concentrations exceeding 1%;
CIR panel says safe in concentrations up to 1%.

†X   m-aminophenol – synthetic; see p-aminophenol.

†X   p-aminophenol – synthetic; used in hair dyes;
mutagen; may cause skin irritation and rashes,
restlessness, convulsions sensitization, asthma if
inhaled; harmful to the liver; not adequately tested;
CIR says safe as used.

XA   Ammonia – synthetic; corrosive; toxic if inhaled;
eye and mucous membrane irritant; can burn eyes
and skin; can cause permanent damage; classified as
hazardous by OSHA; best to avoid all cosmetics
containing ammonia or ammonium salts.

CA   Ammonia water – synthetic; mucous membrane and
eye irritant; may blister and burn skin; toxic when
inhaled; see ammonia.

XA   Ammoniated mercury – synthetic; skin irritant; can
be absorbed through the skin and cause poisoning;
may cause kidney damage; toxic; see ammonia.

XA   Ammonium chloride – synthetic; severe eye and skin
irritant; toxic if ingested in large amounts; may
cause irreversible damage; see ammonia.

X   Ammonium fluoride – synthetic; poison; can be fatal
if swallowed or inhaled; severe irritant; may cause
delayed burning to eyes, skin respiratory tract;
harmful if absorbed by skin; IARC Group 3; not
evaluated by CIR; see fluoride.

X   Ammonium fluorosilicate – synthetic; toxic; can be
fatal if swallowed or inhaled; severe skin, eye,
throat, nose irritant; repeated exposure may cause
fluoride poisoning; not evaluated by CIR; see
fluoride.

CA   Ammonium hydroxide – synthetic; severe skin, eye
and mucous membrane irritant; poison when
swallowed in large amounts; can burn the skin and
cause hair to break; see ammonia.

†CA   Ammonium laureth sulfate – synthetic surfactant;
mild irritant; may be contaminated with carcinogenic
1,4-dioxane; see ethoxylated alcohols, ammonia.

†CA   Ammonium lauroyl sarcosinate – synthetic; CIR panel says safe in "rinse-off" products, safe at 5% concentrations in "leave-on" products, insufficient data to support safety in products which might be inhaled, may cause formation of carcinogens in products containing nitrogen compounds; see ammonia.

†CA   Ammonium lauryl sulfate – synthetic detergent; highly irritating to skin and eyes; causes skin redness and dryness; for brief skin contact only, rinse thoroughly; CIR panel says safe in "rinse-off" products and up to 1% concentrations in "leave-on" products; see ammonia.

†XA   Ammonium thioglycolate – synthetic; cumulative severe skin irritant; may cause burns and blisters; sensitizer; may cause allergic contact dermetitis; highly toxic if inhaled or ingested; has caused death in lab animals; CIR panel says can be used infrequently at concentrations up to 15.4%, but avoid or minimize skin exposure; see ammonia.

XA   Ammonium xylenesulfonate – synthetic; not adequately tested; see ammonia, xylene.

C   Amorphous hydrated silica – respiratory, eye and skin irritant; may be contaminated with crystalline quartz, a carcinogen; IARC Group 3; see external use only; not adequately tested.

C   Amorphous fumed silica – respiratory, eye and skin irritant; may be contaminated with crystalline quartz, a carcinogen; IARC Group 3; see external use only.

C   Amphoteric-2 – synthetic; gentle cleanser; petroleum based; composed of betaines and imidazoles; imidazole is a benzene derivative, but is an inhibitor rather than a toxin; see benzene.

C   Amphoteric-6 – synthetic; a type of sodium lauryl sulfate; see amphoteric-2.

C   Amphoteric-20 – synthetic; see amphoteric-2.

S   Aniba roseodora – see rosewood.

C   Anionic surfactants – may be contaminated with carcinogenic nitrosamines; highly absorbable through skin, even in "rinse-off" products.

*C1   Anise oil – essential oil; antiseptic; anti-inflammatory; helps with menorrhea; may cause dermatitis; avoid in estrogen-dependent cancers, endometriosis; reduces blood pressure; see essential oils.

X   o-anisidine – synthetic; sensitizer; skin irrritant; absorbed through skin; possible carcinogen, IARC Group 2B.

φS   Annatto – plant derived; natural food coloring, antioxidant.

C   Anthanthrene – synthetic; mineral oil contaminant; mutagen; limited evidence of causing cancer in lab animals, but not consistent from study to study; not adequately tested; IARC Group 3.

SA   Anthemis nobilis – essential oil; antiallergenic; antibacterial; anti-inflammatory; astringent; healing for skin; potential sensitive skin irritant.

S   Apricot oil – carrier oil; moisturizing.

C1   Arctium lappa – herb; antibacterial; antidandruff; astringent; avoid if pregnant.

C1   Artemesia dracunculus – plant derived; see tarragon oil.

C1   Artemisia pallens – plant derived; see davana.

C1   Asafetida – plant derived; possible irritant if chemically sensitive; infants and young children should avoid.

C   ASC III – plant derived; safety data not available; see dipalmitoyl hydroxyproline.

*SA   Ascorbic acid – synthetic vitamin C; one component of the vitamin C complex; see nutrient additives; can enhance mineral absorption, can inhibit nitrosamine formation; may be corn based.

†S   Avocado oil – carrier oil.

C   Avobenzone – safety data not available.

X   Azobenzene – synthetic; eye, skin, respiratory irritant; harmful if inhaled, ingested; suspected of causing tumors; derived from nitrobenzene (*see*); genotoxin; EPA rates as probable human carcinogen; Environmental Defense classifies as recognized carcinogen; not adequately tested; IARC Group 3.

C   Azulene – plant derived; not adequately tested; see guaiazulene.

C   Balm – herb; see melissa oil.

CA   Balsam of Peru – plant derived; skin irritant; causes contact dermatitis; sensitizer.

C   Barium –skin, eye and respiratory irritant; never use on broken skin; poisonous if ingested; see external use only.

*C1   Bay oil – essential oil; antiseptic; antifungal; frequent use may cause contact sensitization; possible skin irritant; use cautiously or avoid if pregnant; see essential oils.

CA   Bay rum – plant derived; skin, eye, throat and lung irritant; may cause allergic dermatitis.

†S   Beeswax – natural, from honeycomb; skin irritant; CIR says safe as used.

†C   Bentonite – natural, clay; see magnesium aluminum silicate; CIR says safe as used.

†XA   Benzaldehyde – synthetic; gastrointestinal, mucous membrane, eye and skin irritant; central nervous system depressant; large doses cause convulsions, poisoning; highly toxic; CIR says safe as used.

†XA   Benzalkonium chloride – synthetic; eye and skin irritant; extremely toxic; avoid contact with eyes; CIR says this is safe in concentrations up to .1%; some products contain up to 5%; see quaternary ammonium compounds.

C   Benzamidines – synthetic; may cause contact dermatitis, skin irritation.

X   Benzene – synthetic solvent; petroleum based; skin and mucous membrane irritant; absorbed through skin; photosensitizer; poison if ingested; causes aplastic anemia, poisoning of bone marrow; may cause leukemia; banned in numerous household products; carcinogen, IARC Group 1.

CA   Benzenecarboxylic acid – synthetic; skin irritant, harmful if ingested.

X   Benzethonium chloride – harmful if inhaled, ingested, absorbed through skin; experimental; causes abnormal tissue growth, can be cancerous or benign; quaternary ammonium compound; toxic; suspected endocrine, skin, sense organ toxicant; not adequately tested.

X   Benzo-a-pyrene – synthetic; skin, eye, respiratory irritant; mutagen; recognized carcinogen by Evnironmental Defense; IARC Group 2A; may cause reproductive damage, harm developing fetus, and passed to infant through mother's milk; mineral oil contaminant.

X   Benzo-b-fluroanthene – synthetic; carcinogen, IARC Group 2B; mineral oil contaminant.

C   Benzoates – synthetic; may cause contact dermatitis.

CA   Benzocaine – synthetic; may cause contact dermatitis, has caused oxygen loss in the blood of babies, central nervous system irritability in adults; toxic if ingested.

†CA   Benzoic acid – synthetic; skin irritant, harmful if ingested; implicated in numerous health issues; CIR panel says safe in concentrations up to 5%, insufficient data to support safety in products where exposure involves inhalation.

C   Benzoic acid ethyl ester – synthetic; see ethyl benzoate.

C   Benzoic ether – synthetic; see ethyl benzoate.

CA   Benzoin – synthetic; derived from benzaldehyde; toxic; may cause contact dermatitis.

*S   Benzoin – essential oil; antiseptic, anti-inflammatory; may irritate sensitive skin, cause drowsiness; see essential oils.

*S   Benzoin balm – essential oil; see benzoin.

*S   Benzoin bark – essential oil; see benzoin.

*S   Benzoin gum – essential oil; see benzoin.

*S   Benzoin oil – essential oil; see benzoin.

*S   Benzoin tincture – see benzoin essential oil, ethyl alcohol.

†C   Benzophenone-n (1-12) – synthetic; may cause extreme contact dermatitis, photosensitivity; endocrine disrupter, CIRsays safe as used, except for -7, -10 and -12.

CA   Benzopyrone – can be synthetic or naturally derived; see coumarin.

CA   Benzoyl peroxide – synthetic; corrosive; skin irritant and allergen; toxic if inhaled; IARC Group 3; banned in Europe.

†C   Benzyl alcohol – synthetic; petroleum or coal tar derivative; severe eye, moderate skin and mucous membrane irritant; poison if ingested; CIR panel says safe in concentrations up to 5%, up to 10% in hair dyes, insufficient data to support safety in products where exposure involves inhalation.

CA   Benzyl benzoate – synthetic; skin and eye irritant; on CIR high priority review list.

C   Benzylparaben – synthetic; preservative, may cause mild irritation; insufficient data to support safety according to CIR panel; being re-reviewed by CIR.

*C1   Bergamot oil – essential oil; antibacterial, antiperspirant, astringent, healing properties for hair and skin; may cause contact dermatitis; strong photosensitizer; see essential oils.

ψS   Beta carotene – plant derived; vitamin A precursor; antioxidant.

C   Betaine – synthetic; surfactant; eye, respiratory, skin irritant.

C1   Betula alleghaniensis – essential oil; see birch oil.

CA   Betula pendula – herb; healing to skin; see birch oil.

†XA   BHA – synthetic; may cause contact dermatitis; harmful if ingested; can cause liver and kidney damage, behavioral problems, infertility, weakened immune system, birth defects; possible disrupter; should be avoided by infants, young children, pregnant women, those sensitive to aspirin; possible carcinogen; IARC Group 2B; CIR says safe as used.

†XA   <u>BHT</u> – synthetic; similar to BHA; IARC Group 3; CIR says safe as used.

C   <u>Bilberry</u> – herb; anti-inflammatory; for sensitive skin, gingivitis; may interfere with iron absorption; avoid long-term use; use for 3 weeks periods then take a break.

†S   <u>Biotin</u> – part of the vitamin B complex; important for hair and skin; see nutrient additives; CIR says safe as used.

CA   <u>Birch</u> – herb; see birch oil.

C1   <u>Birch oil</u> – essential oil; anti-inflammatory; antiseptic; avoid if pregnant, epileptic or aspirin sensitive; see methyl salicylate, essential oils.

†C   <u>Bisabolol</u> – essential oil; may be produced synthetically; penetration enhancer; safety data not available; CIR says safe as used; see essential oils.

XA   <u>Bismuth</u> – may cause memory loss, intellectual impairment, nervous system disorders; poison.

φXA   <u>Bismuth citrate</u> – synthetic; poison; absorbed through skin; may cause memory loss, loss of coordination, convulsions; approved for hair dyes only up to .5% concentration; see bismuth.

φXA   <u>Bismuth oxychloride</u> – synthetic; skin irritant; toxic; absorbed through skin; may cause memory loss, loss of coordination, convulsions; see bismuth.

S   <u>Blue mallow</u> – herb; antiallergenic; anti-inflammatory; for sensitive skin.

φXA   <u>Blue No. 1</u> – synthetic; see FD&C Blue No. 1.

XA   <u>Blue No. 1 Lake</u> – synthetic; see FD&C Blue No. 1 Lake.

XA   <u>Blue No. 2</u> – synthetic; see FD&C Blue No. 2.

XA   <u>Blue No. 2 Lake</u> – synthetic; see FD&C Blue No. 2 Lake.

C   <u>Blue No. 99</u> – synthetic; may cause contact dermatitis.

XA   <u>Boranes</u> – synthetic; extremely toxic, may cause contact allergies.

†C   <u>Boric acids</u> – synthetic; toxic; linked to birth defects; topical and internal use have caused poisonings; do not use on infants or damaged skin; not for use by children under age 3; CIR panel says safe up to 5% concentration.

CA   <u>Bornelone</u> – synthetic; may cause contact dermatitis.

S   <u>Boswellia carterii</u> – essential oil; see frankincence oil.

†CA   <u>2-bromo-2-nitropropane-1,3-diol</u> – synthetic; may cause formation of carcinogenic nitrosamines; CIR says $\leq0.1\%$, but should not be used where it's action with amines or amides can cause the formation of nitrosamines or nitrosamides; see bronopol.

|CA   <u>Bronopol</u> – synthetic; toxic; causes contact dermatitis, may cause the formation of carcinogenic nitrosamines; CIR says $\leq0.1\%$, but should not be used where it's action with amines or amides can cause the formation of nitrosamines or nitrosamides; may break down into formaldehyde, an IARC Group 1 carcinogen; see formaldehyde.

φC   <u>Bronze powder</u> – skin, respiratory, digestive irritant; may cause dermatitis; safety data not available.

C1   Burdock – herb; see arctium lappa.

*†C   <u>Butane</u> – synthetic; petroleum derivative; propellant in aerosol products; flammable; may cause drowsiness, asphyxiation; mildly toxic if inhaled; neurotoxic in high doses; CIR says safe as used.

CA   <u>Butanol</u> – synthetic; petroleum derivative; see butyl alcohol.

†CA   <u>Butyl acetate</u> – synthetic; petroleum derivative; toxic; irritant to skin and respiratory tract; central nervous system depressant; CIR says safe as used.

†CA   <u>Butyl alcohol</u> – synthetic; petroleum derivative; skin, eye and respiratory irritant; harmful if absorbed through skin, inhaled, swallowed; may cause liver, kidney damage or adversely affect central nervous system; CIR says safe as used.

X   Butyl Cellosolve – synthetic; petroleum derivative; used in hair dyes; poison; eye and skin irritant; highly absorbable through skin; neurotoxin.

CA   Butyl octadecanoate – synthetic; petroleum derivative; may cause acne.

CA   Butyl stearate – synthetic; respiratory, eye irritant; petroleum derivative; may cause acne; safety data not available.

†XA   Butylated hydroxyanisole – synthetic; petroleum derivative; CIR says safe as used; see BHA.

†XA   Butylated hydroxytoluene – synthetic; petroleum derivative; CIR says safe as used; see BHT.

†CA   Butylene glycol – synthetic solvent; skin and eye irritant; may cause nausea, vomiting and loss of consciousness if ingested; chronic overexposure may cause kidney or liver damage; petroleum derivative; CIR says safe as used.

XA   Butylhydroxyanisol – synthetic; petroleum derivative; carcinogen; see BHA.

†CA   Butylparaben – synthetic; petroleum derivative; skin irritant; associated with numerous of health problems, including contact dermatitis and asthma; strong allergen: currently listed as safe as used, but CIR is re-evaluating safety.

SA   Cacao butter – plant derived; see cocoa butter

X   Cadmium chloride – synthetic; used in hair dyes; carcinogen; ingestion can be fatal; IARC Group 1.

*C1   Cajaput oil – essential oil; antibacterial, anti-inflammatory; skin irritant; not recommended to be used full strength; see essential oils.

*C1   Cajeput oil – see cajaput oil.

*S   Calcium carbonate – derived from limestone; non-hazardous to skin; nontoxic if ingested; dust may irritate skin, eyes, respiratory tract; may constipate.

C   Calcium fluoride – synthetic; toxic; harmful if swallowed or inhaled; may irritate eyes, skin respiratory tract; IARC Group 3; not evaluated by CIR; see fluoride.

C	Calcium monofluorophosphate – synthetic; toxic; harmful if swallowed or inhaled; may irritate eyes, skin respiratory tract; not evaluated by CIR; see fluoride.
C	Calcium oxide – derived from limestone; severe mucous membrane and skin irritant; may cause chemical burns.
S	Calendula – herb; soothes inflammation; nontoxic; minimal skin irritant.
S	Calendula extract see calendula, extract.
S	Calendula officinalis – see calendula.
S	Canadian fleabane – herb with healing properties.
C	Canagium odoratum – see ylang ylang oil.
C	Cananga odorata – essential oil; see ylang ylang oil.
*S	Canarium luzonicum – essential oil; see elemi oil.
†C	Candelilla wax – plant derived; hard, brittle wax, insoluble in water, but soluble in organic solvents such as acetone, benzene or chloroform; slightly soluble in alcohol; may prevent skin from breathing; no known toxicity; CIR says safe as used.
X	Canthanaxin – carotenoid in fungi, shellfish, flamingo feathers; effects on the human body are unknown; not adequately tested.
X	Canthaxanthin – may be derived from flamingo feathers and fungi or synthetic; ingestion can cause night blindness, aplastic anemia; has caused death
C	Canola oil – plant derived, but highly processed; may be genetically modified.
C	Capric acid – plant derived or synthetic; not adequately tested; no known toxicity.
†C	Caprylic /capric triglyceride – synthetic; fractionated coconut oil; highly refined; prolonged skin contact may cause mild irritation, dermatitis or acne; eye irritant; not adequately tested; CIR says safe as used.
C	Capryloyl glycine – capric acid and glycine; amino acid component of elastin and collagen from sunflower seeds and palm; not evaluated by CIR; safety data not available.

φC   Caramel – natural color; not considered hazardous, but long term safety data not available.

C1   Caraway oil – essential oil; promotes wound healing; external use only; caution if pregnant.

C   Carba-mix – synthetic; may cause contact dermatitis.

*C   Carbamide – can be natural, usually synthetic; see urea.

X   3-carbethoxypsoralen – synthetic; phototoxic chemical, may damage DNA and cause mutations, tumors or neoplasms; IARC Group 3.

X   Carbitol – synthetic; toxic; see ethylene glycol.

†CA   Carbomer – synthetic; overexposure may result in mild eye, skin, respiratory and digestive tract irritation; no known toxicity; long-term safety data not available; CIR says safe as used.

†CA   Carbomer 934 – see carbomer.

†CA   Carbomer 940 – see carbomer.

†CA   Carbomer 941 – see carbomer.

CA   Carboxobenzene - synthetic; skin irritant, harmful if ingested.

C   Carboxymethyl cellulose – synthetic; has caused cancer, birth defects, sterility, infertility in animals when ingested; skin toxicity unknown; not evaluated by CIR; not adequately tested.

φCA   Carmine – derived from dried insects; may irritate skin in sensitive individuals; may cause hives; when ingested has caused hives, asthma and anaphylactic shock.

†S   Carnauba wax – natural form derived from Brazilian Wax Palm tree, synthetic derived from petroleum; no known adverse effects; CIR says safe as used.

C   Carotene – synthetic form of pro-vitamin A; may damage retina, reduce production of red blood cells, cause hypersensitivity.

*C   Carrageenan – extracted from red seaweed with powerful alkali solvents; possible carcinogen; native or undegraded carrageenan is IARC Group 3;

degraded carrageenan is IARC Group 2B; not adequately tested.

S   Carrot extract – may cause photo sensitivity.

S   Carrot oil – essential oil; healing to the skin; see essential oils.

C1   Carum carvi – essential oil; see caraway oil.

*C1   Caryophyllus oil – essential oil; see clove oil.

S   Castile soap – made from olive oil.

CA   Castor oil – plant derived; healing properties if cold pressed and cold processed; soothing to the skin; overexposure may cause skin or eye irritation, allergic reaction; long-term use may cause rashes, hypersensitivity.

C1   Cedarwood oil – essential oil; astringent, antifungal, antibacterial; use cautiously or avoid if pregnant; see essential oils.

C1   Cedrus atlantica – essential oil; see cedarwood oil.

C   Cedrus virginiana – essential oil; astringent; antifungal; antibacterial; avoid if pregnant; potentially toxic; use small amounts.

†CA   Cellulose gum –synthetic; overexposure may cause skin, eye, respiratory irritation, allergic dermatitis; mildly toxic if ingested or inhaled; generally considered non toxic; CIR says safe as used.

C1   Centella asiatica – herb; see gotu kola.

CA   Centrurea cyanus – herb; causes photosensitivity.

C   Ceramide 3 – synthetic; moisturizing, nourishing effects; safety data not available.

†CA   Ceresin – synthetic; petroleum derivative; highly refined; bleached and purified ozocerite; long term safety data not found; CIR says safe as used.

†CA   Ceresine⁺ Earth Wax – petroleum derivative; see ceresin.

C   Ceteareth-2-phosphate – synthetic; from cetearyl alcohol and ethylene oxide; may contain carcinogenic contaminants; see ethoxylated alcohols; CIR says should not be used on damaged skin or where N-nitroso compounds could form.

†C   Ceteareth-20 – synthetic; from cetearyl alcohol and ethylene oxide; may contain carcinogenic contaminants; see ethoxylated alcohols; CIR says safe with qualifications - should not be used on damaged skin or where N-nitroso compounds could form.

†S   Cetearyl alcohol – synthetic; may cause contact dermatitis, sensitivity; CIR says safe as used.

S   Cetearyl olivate – synthetic; olive oil derivative.

†C   Ceteth-n – synthetic; may contain dangerous toxic byproducts; CIR says safe as used for -2, -5, -10, -12, -14, -16, -20, -24, -25, -30; see ethoxylated alcohols.

†C   Cetrimonium bromide – synthetic; skin and eye irritant; sensitizer; fatal if swallowed; teratogen in mice; CIR panel says safe as used in "rinse-off" products and up to .25% concentrations in "leave-on" products.

C   Cetyl acetate – synthetic; ester of acetic acid and cetyl alcohol; on CIR high priority list for review.

†CA   Cetyl alcohol – synthetic; may cause skin, eye, respiratory irritation, contact dermatitis; harmful if absorbed through skin; CIR says safe as used.

C   Cetyl stearyl alcohol – synthetic; may cause contact dermatitis.

†CA   Cetylic acid – synthetic; see palmitic acid.

CA   Cetylic alcohol – synthetic; see cetyl alcohol.

X   Chinaldine – synthetic; skin irritant; see quinaldine.

*C1A   Chamomile – herb; anti-inflammatory; may cause allergic contact dermatitis; may interact with certain medications.

*C1A   Chamomile blossom extract – soothing for bruises and inflammation; see chamomile.

*C1A   Chamomile extract – see chamomile, extract.

*C1   Chamomile oil (German) – essential oil; antibacterial, anti-inflammatory, astringent, healing for skin; may irritate sensitive skin; use cautiously if pregnant; see essential oils.

C1 Chamomile oil (Roman) – essential oil; antibacterial, anti-inflammatory, astringent, healing for skin; may irritate sensitive skin; use cautiously if pregnant; see essential oils.

C Chinese anise – essential oil is toxic; herb should be used very sparingly.

C Chinese cinnamon oil – essential oil; avoid if pregnant or fever; see essential oils.

CA Chloracetamide – synthetic; skin, eye and mucous membrane irritant; can be fatal if swallowed; see quaternary ammonium compounds.

X Chloramphenicol – synthetic; antibiotic; may cause eczema; hazardous side effects; probable carcinogen; IARC Group 2A.

†CA Chlorhexidine – synthetic; antimicrobial drug; mouth and tongue irritant; may cause swollen glands on face or neck; may change taste; may stain fillings, teeth or mouth appliances permanantly; may cause hives, itching, swollen face; ingestion may cause nausea, slurred speech, sleepiness; avoid if pregnant or nursing; not for children under 18 years of age or the elderly; may aggravate gum problems, periodontitis; CIR says safe if ≤14%

C Chlorine dioxide – synthetic; poisonous gas that is soluble in water; used in municipal water supplies, cleaning fruits and vegetables, disinfecting poultry, in toothpaste and mouthwash; antimicrobial; classified as a pesticide by the EPA used in cleaning up anthrax contamination; on IARC high-priority list to be evaluated for carcinogenicity.

X Chloroacetamide – synthetic; CIR panel determined this ingredient to be unsafe.

X Chlorofluorocarbons – synthetic; carcinogen; banned in aerosol products in the US.

C Chloromethylisothiazolinone – synthetic; may cause contact dermatitis.

CA 5-chloro-2-methyl-4-iso thiazolin-3-one – synthetic; see isothiazolinones.

CA   <u>5-chloro-3-methyl isothiazolone</u> – synthetic; can cause contact allergies.

X   <u>4-chloro-1,2-phenylenediamine</u> – synthetic; carcinogen.

X   <u>4-chloro-o-phenylenediamine</u> – synthetic; carcinogen; IARC Group 2B.

†X   <u>2-chloro-p-phenylenediamine sulfate</u> – synthetic; carciniogen; contains ammonium salts, CIR says safe a sused; see ammonia.

φS   <u>Chlorophyllin-copper complex</u> – synthetic; see potassium sodium copper chlorophyllin.

C   <u>Chloropromazine group</u> – synthetic; causes phototoxicity.

C   <u>Choleth-n</u> – synthetic; may contain dangerous levels of toxic byproducts; see ethoxylated alcohols.

XA   <u>Chromates</u> – synthetic; may cause contact dermatitis; carcinogen; chromium (IV) compounds, IARC Group1.

C   <u>Chromium</u> – essential trace nutrient in chromium (III) form; too little can cause health problems as well as too much; excess chromium (III) is IARC Group 3.

φCA   <u>Chromium hydroxide green</u> – irritant if inhaled; severe gastrointestinal irritant if ingested; long-term exposure may cause cancer; see external use only; chromium (III), IARC Group 3.

φCA   <u>Chromium oxide greens</u> – eye, skin, respiratory irritant; gastrointestinal irritant if ingested; may harm kidneys, liver; chromium (III), IARC Group 3.

*CA   <u>Cinnamal</u> – synthetic; see cinnamic aldehyde.

*CA   <u>Cinnamaldehyde</u> – synthetic; see cinnamic aldehyde.

CA   <u>Cinnamate</u> – synthetic; may cause skin rashes.

CA   <u>Cinnamic acid</u> – synthetic; see cinoxate.

*CA   <u>Cinnamic aldehyde</u> – synthetic; gastrointestinal, mucous membrane and skin irritant; may cause depigmentation; toxic if swallow large amounts.

*C1   <u>Cinnamomum verum</u> – essential oil; see cinnamon bark oil.

*C1   Cinnamon bark oil – essential oil; anti-bacterial, anti-viral; anti-fungal; skin sensitizer; skin irritant; may cause light sensitivity; causes contact dermatitis; avoid if pregnant; see essential oils.

*C1   Cinnamon oil – essential oil; skin and mucous membrane irritant; causes contact dermatitis; see cinnamon bark oil, essential oils.

C   Cinnamyl aldheyde – synthetic; see cinnamic aldehyde.

CA   Cinoxate synthetic; phototoxic chemical, causes photosensitivity, skin rashes.

†CA   cis-9-octadecenoic acid – synthetic; see oleic acid.

*C1   Cistus ladaniferus – see cistus oil.

*C1   Cistus oil – essential oil; wound healing; antimicrobial; antiseptic; astringent; use cautiously or avoid if pregnant; see essential oils.

C   Citral – plant derived or synthetic; inhibits tumor rejection and wound healing unless Vitamin A is present; causes contact dermatitis; sensitizer.

*C   Citratus – essential oil; see cymbopogon citratus.

*CA   Citric acid – derived from citrus fruit or corn; skin and eye irrtant; that made from other than citrus fruit may contain processed free glutamic acid (MSG); may appear on label as citrate.

*C   Citricidal – plant derived; safe if not contaminated with benzethonium chloride; see grapefruit seed extract.

*C   Citronella – essential oil; antibacterial; anti-fungal; anti-inflammatory; antiseptic; may irritate sensitive skin; skin sensitizer if used frequently; inhalation of pure oil can increase heart rate; use cautiously or avoid if pregnant; see essential oils.

C   Citronellal hydrate – essential oil; see hydroxycitronella.

*S   Citrus aurantifolia – essential oil; see lime oil.

*S   Citrus aurantium – essential oil; see orange oil.

*S   Citrus aurantium bigaradia – essential oil; see neroli oil.

*S   Citrus bergamia essential oil; see bergamot oil.

*S   Citrus lemon – essential oil; see lemon oil.

*S   Citrus limomum – essential oil; see lemon oil.

*S   Citrus nobilis – essential oil; see tangerine oil.

X   Citrus red no. 2 – synthetic; possibly carcinogenic, IARC Group 2B.

*S   Citrus reticulata – essential oil; see mandarin oil.

C1   Civet – essential oil; may irritate chemically sensitive individuals; see essential oils.

*C1   Clary sage oil – essential oil; anti-septic; anti-fungal; astringent; infants and small children should avoid; avoid during/after alcohol consumption; use cautiously or avoid if pregnant; see essential oils.

*C1   Clove oil – essential oil; antibacterial; anti-fungal; anti-infectious; anti-inflammatory; antiseptic; skin irritant; causes contact dermatitis; frequent use may cause contact sensitization; use cautiously or avoid if pregnant; ban proposed for use in astringent products; see essential oils.

XA   Coal tar – coal derivative; skin and eye irritant; phototoxic; carcinogen, IARC Group 1; banned in the European Union; classified as a drug in Canada.

XA   Coal tar derivatives – coal derivative; skin irritant; may cause acne; sensitizer; possible carcinogen; degree of carcenogenicity depends on the specific chemical.

X   Cobalt – heavy metal; skin irritant; possible carcinogen, IARC Group 2B.

X   Cobalt chloride – metal; found in hair dyes; possible carcinogen, IARC Group 2B.

†CA   Cocamide betaine – synthetic; may cause formation of carcinogens in products containing nitrogen compounds.

†CA   Cocamide DEA – synthetic; skin irritant; may cause contact dermatitis, allergies; may cause formation of carcinogens in products containing nitrogen compounds; CIR panel says safe as used in rinse-off products and up to 10% concentrations in leave-on products, but should not be used in products that contain nitrosating agents; see DEA.

†CA   Cocamide diethanolamide – see cocamide DEA.

†CA   Cocamide MEA – synthetic; skin irritant; may cause contact dermatitis, allergies; may cause formation of carcinogens in products containing nitrogen compounds; CIR panel says safe as used in rinse-off products and up to 10% concentrations in leave-on products, but should not be used in products that contain nitrosating agents, and should not be used in aerosol products; see DEA, monoethanolamine.

CA   Cocamide MIPA – synthetic; skin irritant, may cause formation of carcinogens in products containing nitrogen compounds.

†CA   Cocamide monoetanolamine – see cocamide MEA.

CA   Cocamide monoisopropanolamine – see cocamide MIPA.

†CA   Cocamidopropyl betaine – synthetic from coconut oil; may cause contact dermatitis, eyelid dermatitis, eczema, cheilitis; may contain carcinogenic contaminant, nitrosamines; skin sensitizer; see coconut oil; CIR panel says safe as used in rinse-off products, but ≤3% in leave-on products.

CA   Cocamidopropyl Hydroxysultaine – synthetic from coconut oil; see quaternary ammonium compounds; may cause formation of carcinogenic nitrosamines.

φCA   Cochineal extract – see carmine.

SA   Cocoa butter – plant derived; may irritate skin, cause acne, allergic reactions; nontoxic.

†CA   Coco-betaine – see cocamidopropyl betaine.

†CA   Cocobetaine – see cocamidopropyl betaine.

C   Coco-glucoside – synthetic; derived from coconut oil and glucose; mild surfactant; low toxicity; considered safe, but safety data not available; not evaluated by CIR.

†SA   Coconut acid – derived from coconut; mild skin, mucous membrane irritant for some; nontoxic; CIR says safe as used.

†SA   Coconut oil – derived from coconut; skin irritant for some; CIR says safe as used.

†CA   <u>Coconut oil amidopropyl betaine</u> – see cocamidopropyl betaine.

†CA   <u>Cocoyl amide propyldimethyl glycine</u> – see cocamidopropyl betaine.

†C   <u>Cocoyl sarcosine</u> – synthetic; mild cleanser; CIR panel says safe in "rinse-off" products, safe at 5% concentrations in "leave-on" products, insufficient data to determine safety in products which might be inhaled, not to be used in products where N-nitroso compounds could be formed.

C   <u>Coffee extract</u> – natural sunscreen; nervous system and adrenal gland stimulant; harmful in large amounts.

CA   <u>Colamine</u> – synthetic; see ethanolamine.

CA   <u>Collagen</u> – animal protein; allergic reactions common.

CA   <u>Colophony</u> – natural extract; skin irritant.

C   <u>Comfrey</u> – herb; assists wound healing, may cause skin irritation; taken internally may cause liver damage.

C   <u>Comfrey extract</u> – see comfrey.

*C1   <u>Commiphora molmol</u> – essential oil; see myrrh oil.

*C1   <u>Commiphora myrrha</u> – essential oil; see myrrh oil.

φC   <u>Copper powder</u> – dust is eye, mucous membrane irritant; skin irritant with repeated contact; not absorbed through skin; inhalation of large amounts may cause harm; flammable.

*S   <u>Coriander oil</u> – essential oil; analgesic; anti-fungal; anti-bacterial; use sparingly; large doses may induce stupor; see essential oils.

*S   <u>Coriandrum sativum</u> – see coriander oil.

CA   <u>Corn oil</u> – may cause acne; may be genetically modified if not organic.

CA   <u>Cornflower</u> – herb, causes photosensitivity and allergy.

CA   <u>Cornflower distillate</u> – plant extract; phototoxic chemical, causes photosensitivity and allergy.

CA   Cornflower extract – plant extract; phototoxic chemical, causes photosensitivity and allergy; see extract.

CA   Cornstarch – derived from corn; soothing to the skin; may cause skin rash if corn allergy; may cause photosensitivity; may be genetically modified if not organic.

CA   Coumarin – can be synthetic or naturally derived; may cause skin irritation, photosensitivity; toxic; has caused cancer in lab animals; human data not available; not adequately tested; IARC Group 3.

X   Crystalline quartz – carcinogen; IARC Group 1.

X   Crystalline silica – mineral dust; skin, eye and lung irritant; carcinogen, IARC Group 1; most harmful in dry powder form when inhaled.

S   Cucumber – herb; astringent.

S   Cucumis sativus – herb, astringent

CA   Cumarin – see coumarin.

*C1 Cumin oil – essential oil; herbal remedy; photosensitizer; antiviral; toxic if ingested; narcotic in large quantities; use cautiously if pregnant.

C1   Cupressus sempervirens – essential oil; see cypress oil.

X   Cyanide – poison.

C   Cyclohexamide – synthetic; adversely affects skin; toxic if ingested.

†CA Cyclomethicone – synthetic; a silicone fluid; evaporates quickly; not adequately tested; classified as "toxic for reproduction" by the European SCCNFP (Scientific Committee of Cosmetic Products and Non-Food Products intended for Consumers); CIR says safe as used.

C   Cyclopentasiloxane – synthetic; a silicone fluid not readily absorbed by the skin; see cyclomethicone; safety data not available; not adequately tested; not evaluated by CIR; see silicones.

*S   Cymbopogon citratus – essential oil; see lemongrass oil.

*S   Cymbopogon flexuosis – essential oil; see lemongrass oil.

*S   Cymbopogon martini – essential oil; see palmarosa oil.

*C1   Cymbopogon nardus – essential oil; see citronella.

C1   Cypress oil – essential oil; astringent, insect repellant, deodorant; use cautiously or avoid if pregnant; see essential oils.

φXA   D&C Blue No. 4 – synthetic coal tar dye; potential carcinogen; see external use only, D&C Colors, coal tar.

XA   D&C Blue No. 4 Lake – synthetic coal tar dye; may contain aluminum; see D&C Blue No. 4, aluminum powder.

φXA   D&C Brown No. 1 – synthetic azo dye; mucous membrane and skin irritant; if absorbed into the body, can deplete oxygen and cause death; see external use only, D&C Colors.

φX   D&C Colors – colors considered safe by the FDA for drugs and cosmetics, but not for food; disregards permeability of the skin which allows these substances to be absorbed into the body; most of the colors are derived from coal tar and must be certified by the FDA not to contain more than 20ppm of lead and arsenic; certification does not address any harmful effects these colors may have on the body; most coal tar colors are potential carcinogens, may contain carcinogenic contaminants, and cause allergic reactions.

φXA   D&C Green No. 5 – synthetic coal tar color; skin irritant; low toxicity; see D&C Colors; coal tar.

XA   D&C Green No. 5 Lake – synthetic coal tar color; may contain aluminum; see D&C Green No. 5, aluminum powder.

φXA   D&C Green No. 6 – synthetic coal tar dye; skin irritant; potential carcinogen; see external use only, D&C Colors, coal tar.

XA   **D&C Green No. 6 Lake** – synthetic coal tar dye; may contain aluminum; see D&C Green No. 6, aluminum powder.

φXA   **D&C Green No. 8** – synthetic pyrene color; potentially carcinogenic; see external use only, D&C Colors.

φXA   **D&C Orange No. 4** – synthetic monoazo dye; potential carcinogen; see external use only, D&C Colors.

XA   **D&C Orange No. 4 Lake** – synthetic monoazo dye; may contain aluminum; see D&C Orange No. 4, aluminum powder.

φXA   **D&C Orange No. 5** – synthetic coal tar dye; may cause cheilitis; carcinogen; see external use only, D&C Colors.

XA   **D&C Orange No. 5 Lake** – synthetic coal tar dye; may contain aluminum; see D&C Orange No. 5, aluminum powder.

φXA   **D&C Orange No. 10** – synthetic coal tar dye; possible photosensitizer, mutagen; see external use only, D&C Colors.

XA   **D&C Orange No. 10 Lake** – synthetic coal tar dye; may contain aluminum; see D&C Orange No. 10, aluminum powder.

φXA   **D&C Orange No. 11** – synthetic coal tar dye; see external use only, D&C Colors; coal tar.

XA   **D&C Orange No. 11 Lake** – synthetic coal tar dye; may contain aluminum; see D&C Orange No. 11, aluminum powder.

X   **D&C Orange No. 17** – carcinogen; banned.

φXA   **D&C Red No. 6** –synthetic monoazo color; may cause acne; potential carcinogen; see D&C Colors, external use only.

XA   **D&C Red No. 6 Lake** – synthetic monoazo color; may contain aluminum; see D&C Red No. 6, aluminum powder.

φXA   D&C Red No. 7 – synthetic monoazo color; may
       cause acne; potential carcinogen; see D&C Colors,
       external use only.

XA   D&C Red No. 7 Lake – synthetic monoazo color;
       may contain aluminum; see D&C Red No. 7,
       aluminum powder.

X   D&C Red No. 9 – synthetic; has caused cancer in lab
       animals; no human data available; IARC Group 3;
       banned.

φXA   D&C Red No. 17 – synthetic; may cause acne;
       carcinogen; see external use only, D&C Colors,
       external use only.

XA   D&C Red No. 17 Lake – synthetic; may contain
       aluminum; see D&C Red No. 17, aluminum powder.

X   D&C Red No. 19 – synthetic; carcinogen; banned.

φXA   D&C Red No. 21 – synthetic coal tar color; may
       cause acne, cheilitis, photosensitivity; possible
       mutagen; see D&C Colors, external use only.

XA   D&C Red No. 21 Lake – synthetic coal tar color;
       may contain aluminum; see D&C Red No. 21,
       aluminum powder.

φXA   D&C Red No. 22 – synthetic coal tar color; potential
       carcinogen; may cause acne; see D&C Colors,
       external use only, coal tar.

XA   D&C Red No. 22 Lake – synthetic coal tar color;
       may contain aluminum; see D&C Red No. 22,
       aluminum powder.

φXA   D&C Red No. 27 – synthetic coal tar color; possible
       carcinogen; may cause acne, cheilitis; see D&C
       Colors, external use only, coal tar.

XA   D&C Red No. 27 Lake – synthetic coal tar color;
       may contain aluminum; see D&C Red No. 27,
       aluminum powder.

φXA   D&C Red No. 28 – synthetic coal tar color; possible
       carcinogen; may cause acne; see D&C Colors,
       external use only, coal tar.

XA   <u>D&C Red No. 28 Lake</u> – synthetic coal tar color; may contain aluminum; see D&C Red No. 28, aluminum powder.

φCA   <u>D&C Red No. 30</u> – synthetic indigoid color; may cause acne; see D&C Colors, external use only.

CA   <u>D&C Red No. 30 Lake</u> – synthetic indigoid color; may contain aluminum; see D&C Red No. 30, aluminum powder.

φXA   <u>D&C Red No. 31</u> – synthetic monoazo color; potential carcinogen; may cause acne; see external use only, D&C Colors.

XA   <u>D&C Red No. 31 Lake</u> – synthetic monoazo color; may contain aluminum; see D&C Red No. 31, aluminum powder.

φXA   <u>D&C Red No. 33</u> synthetic monoazo color; potential carcinogen; may cause acne; may contain carcinogenic impurities; see external use only, D&C Colors.

XA   <u>D&C Red No. 33 Lake</u> – synthetic monoazo color; may contain aluminum; may contain carcinogenic impurities; see D&C Red No. 33, aluminum powder.

φXA   <u>D&C Red No. 34</u> – synthetic monoazo color; potential carcinogen; may cause acne; see external use only, D&C Colors.

XA   <u>D&C Red No. 34 Lake</u> – synthetic monoazo color; may contain aluminum; see D&C Red No. 34, aluminum powder.

φXA   <u>D&C Red No. 36</u> – synthetic monoazo color; potential carcinogen; may cause acne, dermatitis; see external use only, D&C Colors.

XA   <u>D&C Red No. 36 Lake</u> – synthetic monoazo color; may contain aluminum; see D&C Red No. 36, aluminum powder.

φXA   <u>D&C Violet No. 2</u> – synthetic coal tar dye; skin irritant; has caused tumors in rats; see external use only, D&C Colors, coal tar.

XA   <u>D&C Violet No. 2 Lake</u> – synthetic coal tar dye; may contain aluminum; see D&C Violet No. 2, aluminum powder.

φXA   <u>D&C Yellow No. 7</u> – synthetic coal tar dye; mutagen; see external use only, D&C Colors, fluoresceins.

XA   <u>D&C Yellow No. 7 Lake</u> – synthetic coal tar dye; may contain aluminum; see D&C Yellow No. 7, aluminum powder.

φXA   <u>D&C Yellow No. 8</u> – synthetic coal tar dye; potential carcinogen; see external use only, D&C Colors; coal tar.

XA   <u>D&C Yellow No. 8 Lake</u> – synthetic coal tar dye; may contain aluminum; see D&C Yellow No. 8, aluminum powder.

φXA   <u>D&C Yellow No. 10</u> – synthetic coal tar dye; skin irritant; potential carcinogen; see D&C Colors, external use only, coal tar.

XA   <u>D&C Yellow No. 10 Lake</u> – synthetic coal tar dye; may contain aluminum; see D&C Yellow No. 10, aluminum powder.

φXA   <u>D&C Yellow No. 11</u> – synthetic coal tar dye; skin irritant; potential carcinogen; see external use only, D&C Colors, coal tar.

S   <u>Daucus carota</u> – essential oil; see carrot oil.

C1   <u>Davana oil</u> – essential oil; use cautiously or avoid if pregnant.

X   <u>DBP</u> – synthetic; used in nail polish; see phthalates; banned in Europe.

†CA   <u>DEA</u> – synthetic; mucous membrane, eye and skin irritant; absorbed through skin; carcinogen in mice; may cause formation of carcinogens with nitrogen containing compounds; may contain nitrosamine contaminants not listed on the label; no data on humans available; IARC Group 3; not adequately tested; CIR panel says safe up to 5% concentration in "rinse-off" products only.

CA   DEA cetyl phosphate – synthetic; may cause formation of carcinogens; see DEA.

CA   DEA dihydroxypalmityl phosphate – synthetic; may cause formation of carcinogens; see DEA.

CA   DEA lauryl sulfate – synthetic; irritant; may cause formation of carcinogens; contains ammonium salts; see DEA, ammonia.

CA   DEA methoxycinnamate – synthetic; phototoxic chemical, in sunlight may cause formation of carcinogenic nitrosamines; see DEA.

CA   Decyl glucoside –synthetic surfactant; no known skin toxicity; non-irritating; assumed safe, mild and gentle, but safety data not available; may cause contact allergy; not evaluated by CIR.

†S   Decyl oleate –synthetic surfactant; may cause acne; CIR says safe as used.

C   Decyl polyglucose – synthetic surfactant; derived from corn and coconut; gentle; no known adverse effects; assumed safe, mild and gentle, but safety data not available; not evaluated by CIR.

C   DEET – synthetic; poison if ingested; eye and mucous membrane irritant.

X   DEHP – synthetic; used in perfumes; see phthalates, banned in Europe.

C   Denatured alcohol – synthetic; severe skin irritant; poisonous; inhalation may cause headaches, dizziness, difficulty breathing; ingestion may cause headaches, dizziness, blindness, coma, death.

S   Deionized water

*Cl   Delphinensis – essential oil; see lavandin.

X   DEP – synthetic; used in perfumes; see phthalates.

X   Diamine – synthetic; skin and eye irritant; carcinogen; banned in Europe.

X   2,4-diaminoanisol – synthetic; carcinogen, IARC Group 2B; mutagen, may cause genetic damage.

X   2,5-diaminoanisol – synthetic; mutagen, may cause genetic damage.

X   2,4-diaminoanisole sulfate – synthetic; carcinogen,
       mutagen, may cause genetic damage; contains
       ammonium salts, see ammonia.
X   m-diaminobenzene – synthetic; see m-
       phenylenediamine.
C   Diatomaceous earth – amorphous silica; IARC
       Group 3.
XA   1,2-diaminoethane – synthetic; ee ethylenediamine.
X   2,4-diaminotoluene – synthetic; causes dermatitis,
       sensitization; possible carcinogen, IARC Group 2B;
       mutagen; may cause genetic damage; causes
       reproductive toxicity.
CA   Diammonium dithiodiglycolate – synthetic; skin
       irritant.
†C   Diazolidinyl urea – synthetic; preservative; skin
       irritant; may cause dermatitis; may release
       formaldehyde; CIR panel says safe up to .5%
       concentration; see formaldehyde.
CA   Dibromocyanobutane – synthetic; skin irritant;
       preservative.
C   1,2-dibromo-2,4-dicyanobutane – synthetic; causes
       eczema.
X   Dibutyl phthalate – synthetic; see phthalates.
X   Dichlorobenzyl alcohol – synthetic; not tested for
       safety; see benzyl alcohol.
X   1,2-dichloroethane – synthetic; carcinogen, IARC
       Group 2B.
XA   Dichlorophen – synthetic; toxic; skin and eye
       irritant; may cause diarrhea and cramps; potent
       allergen.
XA   Dichlorophene – synthetic; see dichlorophen.
†CA   Diethanolamine – synthetic; see DEA.
C   Diethyl maleate – synthetic; causes contact
       dermatitis.
X   1,4-diethylene dioxide – synthetic; see 1,4-dioxane.
X   Diethylene ether – synthetic; see 1,4-dioxane.
X   Diethylene glycol – synthetic; toxic; absorbs through
       skin; hazardous if used on large areas of the body;
       ingestion can be fatal.

X   Diethylene oxide – synthetic; see 1,4-dioxane.

X   Diethylnitrosamine – synthetic; carcinogen.

C   Digalloyl trioleate – synthetic; phototoxic chemical, causes photosensitivity.

C   5,7-dihydroxy-4-methyl coumarin – synthetic; sensitizes skin.

φCA   Dihydroxyacetone – synthetic; skin irritant; has caused death when large doses injected into rats; see external use only.

C   5,7-dihydroxycoumarin – synthetic; sensitizes skin.

X   Diisopropanolnitrosamine – synthetic; carcinogen; contains ammonium salts, see ammonia.

C   Dimethicon – synthetic; has caused mutations and tumors in lab animals.

†CA   Dimethicone – synthetic; irritant; use on skin may cause internal problems; low toxicity; CIR says safe as used in cosmetics; see silicones.

†CA   Dimethicone copolyol – synthetic; safer version of dimethicone; contains PEG; may contain harmful contaminants; see PEG: CIR says safe as used in cosmetics.

†CA   Dimethicone PEG-6 Acetate – synthetic; see dimethicone copolyol.

†CA   Dimethicone PEG-7 Phosphate – synthetic; see dimethicone copolyol.

†CA   Dimethicone PEG-8 Adipate – synthetic; see dimethicone copolyol.

†CA   Dimethicone PEG-8 Benzoate – synthetic; see dimethicone copolyol.

†CA   Dimethicone PEG-10 Phosphate – synthetic; see dimethicone copolyol.

†CA   Dimethicone PEG/PPG-7/4 Phosphate – synthetic; see dimethicone copolyol.

†CA   Dimethicone PEG/PPG-12/4 Phosphate – synthetic; see dimethicone copolyol.

†CA   Dimethicone PEG/PPG-20/23 Benzoate – synthetic; see dimethicone copolyol.

X   Dimethyl Ether – synthetic; eye, skin, musous membrane irritant; may cause dermatitis, drowsiness, dizziness, frostbite; harmful amounts may be absorbed through skin; inhalation may depress central nervous system, cause respiratory failure, unconsciousness; on CIR high priority review list.

CA 3,7-dimethyl-7-hydroxyoctenal –synthetic or synthetic; see hydroxycitronella.

C 3,7-dimethyl-1,6-octadien-3-ol – essential oil; see linalool.

CA Dimethyl lauramine – synthetic; may cause formation of carcinogens; insufficient data to support safety according to CIR panel.

CA Dimethyl stearamine – synthetic; may cause formation of carcinogens; insufficient data to support safety according to CIR panel.

X Dimethylamine – synthetic; severe eye, skin, mucous membrane irritant; absorbed through skin; may be fatal if inhaled; see ammonia.

X Dimethylnitrosamine – synthetic; carcinogen; easily absorbed through skin; contains ammonium salt, see ammonia.

X Dioctyl phthalate – synthetic; eye, skin and mucous membrane irritant; carcinogen; central nervous system depressant.

*X Dioctyl sodium sulfosuccinate – synthetic; see sodiumsulfosuccinate.

*X Dioctyl sulfosuccinate sodium – synthetic; see sodiumsulfosuccinate.

C Dioctyl sebacate – synthetic; skin and eye irritant; inhalation may cause nausea, respiratory tract irritation; flammable.

X Dioxane – synthetic; industrial poison; carcinogen, IARC Group 2B.

X 1,4-dioxane – synthetic; carcinogen, IARC Group 2B; found in 40% of cosmetics; absorbed through skin; toxic if inhaled; may be removed during processing by vacuum stripping, but product labels do not give adequate information to determine if the product is contaminated.

C   Dioxybenzone – synthetic; see benzophenone.

X   Dioxyethylene ether – synthetic; see 1,4-dioxane.

C   Dipalmitoyl hydroxyproline – plant derived lipid amino acid complex naturally present in skin; safety data not available; not evaluated by CIR.

C   Dipalmitoylethyldimonium Chloride – synthetic; see quaternary ammonium compounds; no safety information available; not adequately tested.

†C   Diphenylketone – synthetic; see benzophenone.

X   Direct black 38 – synthetic; carcinogen.

X   Direct blue 6 – synthetic; carcinogen.

X   Diresorcinolphthalein – synthetic; see fluoresceins.

†CA   Disodium EDTA – synthetic; may cause formation of carcinogens in products containing nitrogen compounds; mucous membrane, eye and skin irritant; may cause asthma, kidney damage: penetration enhancer; CIR says safe as used.

φCA   Disodium EDTA-copper – synthetic; approved for shampoo only; see disodium EDTA

C   Disodium laureth sulfosuccinate – synthetic surfactant; may contain toxic byproducts; see ethoxylated alcohols.

C   Disodium lauryl sulfosuccinate – synthetic surfactant; not adequately tested; not evaluated by CIR.

C   Disodium oleamido PEG – synthetic; may contain toxic byproducts; see ethoxylated alcohols.

S   Disodium phosphate – synthetic; skin and eye irritant.

CA   Disodium salt – synthetic; see disodium EDTA.

X   DM hydantoin – synthetic; methanol derivative; has caused cancer in lab animals; may cause contact dermatitis; on CIR high priority list for review.

X   DMD hydantoin – synthetic; preservative; may contain formaldehyde.

†X   DMDM hydantoin – synthetic; may cause dermatitis; may contain formaldehyde; hydantoin has caused cancer in rats; CIR says safe as used; see formaldehyde.

X   DMP – synthetic; used in perfumes; see phthalates.

C   1-dodecanol – synthetic; see lauryl alcohol.

C   Dodecyl alcohol – synthetic; see lauryl alcohol.

XA   p-dohydroxybenzene – synthetic; see hydroquinone.

CA   Dowicil – synthetic; preservative; may cause allergic reactions.

C   DPHP – see dipalmitoyl hydroxyproline.

CA   Dyes – synthetic; soluble colors, usually petroleum based; see coal tar derivatives, hair dyes.

S   Echinacea – herb; heals damaged skin; immune system stimulant.

S   Echinacea angustifolia – see echinacea.

†CA   EDTA – synthetic; CIR says says safe as used; see disodium EDTA.

C   Elastin – a protein in the skin; elastin in cosmetics is derived from animals and cannot changed the elasticity of human skin; does not penetrate the skin; may prevent the skin from breathing; not adequately tested.

*S   Elemi oil – essential oil; antiseptic; aids allergic rashes, chapped skin.

C   EMA – see ethyl methacrylate.

C   Emulsifying wax – synthetic; chemical mixture of fatty alcohols and emulsifiers; potential skin irritant; may cause contact dermatitis; see emulsifying wax NF.

†C   Emulsifying wax NF – synthetic; chemical mixture of fatty alcohols and emulsifiers, such as cetearyl alcohol, polysorbate 60, PEG-150 stearate, steareth-20; potential skin irritant; may cause contact dermatitis; may contain ingredients with carcinogenic contaminants; CIR says safe as used.

X   Epoxyethane – synthetic; see ethylene oxide.

C1   Equisetum arvense – herb; see horse tail.

XA   Erythrosine Potassium – synthetic; see coal tar derivatives.

XA   Erythrosine Sodium – synthetic; see coal tar derivatives.

X   Essence of mirabane – synthetic; see nitrobenzene.

C   Essence of Niobe – synthetic; see ethyl benzoate.

C   Essential oils – properly extracted for highest purity and used knowledgeably, essential oils have great therapeutic benefit; used as an ingredient in cosmetics and personal care products, most essential oils are safe; used full strength, cautions may be advised; pure essential oils do not cause allergic reactions; reactions to pure essential oils are detox reactions. If synthetics are added, the effect may be altered; if solvent or heat extracted, they are highly refined and lose beneficial properties; toxic solvent extraction contaminants may remain in the finished product; all absolutes are solvent extracted. Different brands of oils vary in quality, effectiveness and safety; 95% of oils sold are altered and are perfume or food grade, not pure; if uncertain if synthetics are added, more caution is advised. Consult your physician if pregnant or other health issues.

XA   1,2-ethanediol – synthetic; see ethylene glycol.

C   Ethanol – derived from fermented carbohydrates, starch and sugar; see ethyl alcohol.

†CA   Ethanolamine – synthetic; severe nose, throat, eye and skin irritant; absorbed through skin; central nervous system depressant; may cause kidney, liver damage; may cause formation of carcinogens in products containing nitrogen compounds; mutagen; CIR says safe for rinse-off products, NOT for leave-on products.

CA   Ethanolamines – synthetic; see ethanolamine.

C   Ether – synthetic; skin irritant; may cause central nervous system depression if inhaled or ingested.

C   Ethers – synthetic; skin irritant; may cause central nervous system depression if inhaled or ingested.

X   Ethoxyethanol – synthetic; CIR panel determined this ingredient to be unsafe.

X   Ethoxyethanol acetate – synthetic; CIR panel determined this ingredient to be unsafe.

CA 2-ethoxyethyl-p-methoxy cinnamate – synthetic; phototoxic chemical, causes photosensitivity, skin rashes.

C Ethoxylated alcohols – synthetic; may contain carcinogenic contaminant, 1,4-dioxane, which is rapidly absorbed through the skin; may be removed during processing by vacuum stripping, but product labels do not give adequate information to determine if the product is contaminated.

CA Ethoxylated lanolins – synthetic; skin irritant; may cause acne; may contain harmful amounts of toxic byproducts.

†C Ethyl acetate – synthetic; skin irritant; may cause liver, kidney damage, central nervous system depression; CIR says safe as used.

C Ethyl alcohol – synthetic solvent; drying to skin and hair; may cause contact dermatitis; eye irritant; carcinogen and mutagen if swallowed.

C Ethyl benzenecarboxylate – see ethyl benzoate.

C Ethyl benzoate – synthetic; eye and skin irritant; toxic if swallow large amounts.

†C Ethyl ester of PVM/MA copolymer – synthetic; toxic if inhaled; long term safety data not available; CIR panel says safe in neutralized form in cosmetics.

C Ethyl methacrylate – synthetic; eye and skin irritant; inhalation can cause headaches, dizziness, nausea; may also cause asthma and allergic reactions.

CA Ethyl-p-aminobenzoate – synthetic; may cause contact dermatitis, has caused oxygen loss in the blood of babies, central nervous system irritability in adults.

CA Ethyl-p-hydroxybenzoate – synthetic; preservative; skin irritant; strong allergen; toxic.

XA Ethylene alcohol – synthetic; see ethylene glycol.

XA Ethylene glycol – synthetic; derived from petroleum; skin and respiratory irritant; severe eye irritant; harmful if absorbed through skin, ingested or inhaled; toxic; can cause contact dermatitis; may cause kidney, liver, respiratory problems, death; mutagen; neurotoxin; reproductive hazard.

X   Ethylene oxide – synthetic; skin and eye irritant; may cause kidney damage; harmful if swallowed; carcinogen IARC Group 1; may cause inheritable genetic damage.

XA   Ethylenediamine – synthetic; skin and eye irritant, sensitizer; may cause asthma; toxic if inhaled or absorbed through skin.

CA   Ethylenediaminetetraacetic acid – synthetic; see disodium EDTA.

C   Ethylhexyl methoxycinnamate – synthetic; may cause stinging sensation; skin and eye irritant; toxological data not available

†CA   Ethylparaben – synthetic; associated with numerous of health problems, including contact dermatitis and asthma; strong allergen; endocrine disrupter; see ethyl-p-hydroxybenzoate: CIR says safe as used, but CIR is re-evaluating safety.

*C1   Eucalyptus citriodora – essential oil; see eucalyptus oil (lemon scented).

*C1   Eucalyptus globulus – essential oil, antibacterial, anti-inflammatory, insect repellant; not for small children; avoid if epilepsy, high blood pressure, pregnant; see essential oils.

*C1   Eucalyptus oil – essential oil; antibacterial, anti-inflammatory, insect repellant; not for small children; avoid if epilepsy, high blood pressure, pregnant; see essential oils.

*C1   Eucalyptus oil (lemon scented) – essential oil; antibacterial; anti-fungal; anti-infectious; anti-inflammatory; antiseptic; frequent use may cause contact sensitization; see essential oils.

*C1   Eugenia caryophyllus – essential oil; see clove oil.

*CA   Eugenol – synthetic; skin irritant; causes contact dermatitis; mutagen; toxic if swallowed; limited evidence of carcenogenicity in lab animals; no human data available; not adequately tested; IARC Group 3.

φC   External use only – the FDA has approved, as safe, some colorants "for external use only" disregarding the fact that substances put on the skin can be absorbed into the body. If these substances are harmful when ingested, they will still be harmful when absorbed into the body.

φX   Ext. D&C Colors – colors considered safe by the FDA for drugs and cosmetics used externally on the skin, but not on the mucous membranes or for food; disregards permeability of the skin which allows these substances to be absorbed into the body; most of the colors are derived from coal tar and must be certified by the FDA not to contain more than 20ppm of lead and arsenic; certification does not address any harmful effects these colors may have on the body; most coal tar colors are potential carcinogens, may contain carcinogenic contaminants and cause allergic reactions.

φXA   Ext. D&C Violet No. 2 – synthetic; coal tar color; see D&C Violet No. 2; see external use only, Ext. D&C Colors; coal tar.

φXA   Ext. D&C Yellow No. 7 – synthetic; coal tar color; skin irritant; potential carcinogen; see external use only, Ext. D&C Colors; coal tar.

XA   Ext. D&C Yellow No. 7 Lake – synthetic; may contain aluminum; see Ext. D&C Yellow No. 7, aluminum powder.

C   Extract – extraction may be by cold or hot hydraulic pressing or by organic solvents; solvent extraction requires the solvent to be refined out and may leave toxic contaminant residue in the extract; hot pressing and solvent extraction cause loss of beneficial substances and are highly refined; only cold pressing preserves beneficial ingredients.

†S   Extract of aloe vera – herb; see aloe, extract.

C   Extract of balm mint – herb; no known toxicity; see extract.

C1   Extract of burdock – herb; see burdock, extract.

S   Extract of calendula – herb; see calendula, extract.

SA   Extract of chamomile – herb; see chamomile, extract.

C   Extract of coltsfoot – herb; avoid excess or long term use; avoid while pregnant and nursing; large doses may cause liver damage; see extract.

C   Extract of comfrey – herb; see comfrey, extract.

S   Extract of cucumber – herb; see extract.

C   Extract of grapefruit – herb; see grapefruit seed extract.

C1   Extract of horsetail – herb; see horsetail, extract.

C1A   Extract of hypericum – herb; see hypericum perforatum, extract.

C1A   Extract of ivy – herb; see ivy extract, extract.

C1A   Extract of matricaria – herb; see chamomile, extract.

S   Extract of orchid – plant extract; no known safety issues when used as recommended; see extract.

C1   Extract of sambucus – herb; diuretic; avoid if pregnant; only sambucus nigra is safe; sambucus ebulus and sambucus racemosa are toxic; see extract.

C   Extract of stinging nettle – herb; see nettle, extract.

C   Extract of valerian – herb; see valerian oil, extract.

C1   Extract of yarrow – herb; see yarrow oil, extract.

C   Fatty acids – plant or animal derived; essential fatty acids are necessary for good health; fatty acids used in toiletries are generally synthetic oleochemicals; may also be derived from petrochemicals; may contain trans fats; a German study found carcinogenic contaminants.

C   Fatty acid esters – synthetic; derived from oleochemicals; see fatty acids; no known toxicity.

CA   Fatty alcohols – synthetic; derived from oleochemicals; may also be derived from petrochemicals; may cause allergic reaction, skin irritation; low toxicity; may contain trans fats.

C   Fatty amine oxides – synthetic; may be contaminated with carcinogens.

φXA   FD&C Blue No. 1 – synthetic; coal tar dye; carcinogen; see FD&C Colors, coal tar.

XA   <u>FD&C Blue No. 1 Lake</u> – synthetic; coal tar dye; carcinogen; may contain aluminum; see FD&C Colors, aluminum powder.

XA   <u>FD&C Blue No. 2</u> – synthetic; coal tar dye; potential carcinogen; see FD&C Colors; coal tar.

XA   <u>FD&C Blue No. 2 Lake</u> – synthetic; coal tar dye; potential carcinogen; may contain aluminum; see FD&C Colors, aluminum powder.

ϕX   <u>FD&C Colors</u> – synthetic; colors considered safe by the FDA for use in food, drugs and cosmetics; most of the colors are derived from coal tar and must be certified by the FDA not to contain more than 10ppm of lead and arsenic; certification does not address any harmful effects these colors may have on the body; most coal tar colors are potential carcinogens, may contain carcinogenic contaminants, and cause allergic reactions.

ϕXA   <u>FD&C Green No. 3</u> – synthetic; carcinogen; see FD&C Colors.

XA   <u>FD&C Green No. 3 Lake</u> – synthetic; may contain aluminum; see FD&C Green No. 3, aluminum powder.

XA   <u>FD&C Red No. 3</u> – synthetic; carcinogen, color derived from coal tar; banned for cosmetics and drugs used externally; still approved for use in foods and drugs taken internally; see FD&C Colors, coal tar.

ϕXA   <u>FD&C Red No. 4</u> – synthetic; coal tar dye; causes atrophied adrenal glands and bladder polyps in animals, banned in food and drugs, but allowed in cosmetics; see external use only, FD&C Colors, coal tar.

XA   <u>FD&C Red No. 4 Lake</u> – synthetic; may contain aluminum; see FD&C Red No. 4, aluminum powder.

ϕXA   <u>FD&C Red No. 40</u> – synthetic; monoazo color; suspected carcinogen; may be contaminated with carcinogens; see FD&C Colors.

φXA FD&C Red No. 40 Aluminum Lake – synthetic; may be contaminated with a carcinogen; see FD&C Colors, aluminum powder.

φXA FD&C Yellow No. 5 – synthetic; coal tar dye; potential carcinogen; may contain carcinogenic contaminants; aspirin sensitive individuals may develop life-threatening symptoms; see FD&C Colors.

XA FD&C Yellow No. 5 Lake – synthetic; may contain aluminum; see FD&C Yellow No. 5, aluminum powder.

φXA FD&C Yellow No. 6 – synthetic; coal tar dye; potential carcinogen; may contain carcinogenic contaminants; see FD&C Colors, coal tar.

XA FD&C Yellow No. 6 Lake – synthetic; may contain aluminum; see FD&C Yellow No. 6, aluminum powder.

*C1 Fennel oil – essential oil; skin irritant; antiseptic; frequent use may cause contact sentization; avoid if kidney problems; use cautiously or avoid if pregnant or epileptic; see essential oils.

φC Ferric ammonium ferrocyanide – synthetic; see external use only.

φC Ferric ferrocyanide – synthetic; see external use only.

C1 Ferula gummose – essential oil; see galbanum.

S Fir oil – essential oil; may offer therapeutic benefit; irritant to sensitive skin.

S Flavonoids – herbs; tone skin; strengthen capillaries.

SA Flaxseed oil – plant derived; see linseed oil.

X Fluoranthene – synthetic; mutagen; not adequately tested for carcinogenic effects; IARC Group 3.

X Fluoresceins – synthetic; may damage DNA and cause mutations, tumors or neoplasms.

X Fluoride – synthetic; skin, eye, nose, throat irritant; poison; causes premature aging, weakening of the immune system, mottling of the teeth, anemia, joint stiffness, calcified ligaments, genetic damage; IARC Group 3.

*C1   <u>Foeniculum vulgare</u> – essential oil; see fennel oil.

†XA   <u>Formaldehyde</u> – synthetic; carcinogen, IARC Group 1, mutagen; neurotoxin; sensitizer; eye and skin irritant; may trigger asthma; poison if swallowed; CIR panel says safe up to .2% free formaldehyde, not safe in aerosol products; banned in Japan and Europe.

XA   <u>Formalin</u> – synthetic; see formaldehyde.

XA   <u>Formic aldehyde</u> – synthetic; see formaldehyde.

XA   <u>Formol</u> – synthetic; see formaldehyde.

CA   <u>Fragrance</u> – synthetic; may irritate skin; may cause cheilitis, headaches, dizziness, coughing, vomiting, skin discoloration; manufacturers are not required to disclose chemicals used for fragrance; mostly derived from petroleum; some hazardous chemicals found in fragrance include benzyl chloride, ethyl alcohol, methylene chloride, methyl ethyl ketone, methyl isobutyl ketone, phthalates and toluene; a single fragrance may contain hundreds of different chemicals; may contain carcinogens.

*S   <u>Frankincense oil</u> – essential oil; antiseptic; antidepressant; immune-stimulant; see essential oils.

†C   <u>Fruit acids</u> – synthetic; see alpha hydroxy acids.

C   <u>Fumaric acid</u> – natural or synthetic; eye, skin irritant; toxic on skin contact or ingestion; on CIR high priority review list.

X   <u>Furocoumarines</u> – synthetic; phototoxic chemical; may damage DNA and cause mutations, tumors or neoplasms.

X   <u>Furocoumarin-plus-UVA</u> – synthetic; phototoxic chemical; may damage DNA and cause mutations, tumors or neoplasms.

S   <u>Galacturonic acid</u> – plant derived; constituent of plant pectins found in fruits and vegetables.

C1   <u>Galbanum</u> – essential oil; antiseptic; anti-inflammatory; potential irritant for the chemically sensitive; avoid during first trimester of pregnancy; see essential oils.

C1   Garlic – herb; antibacterial; fresh juice may cause burns; avoid during pregnancy.

C1   Garlic oil – see garlic.

SA   Geraniol – occurs naturally in fruits, herbs and essential oils; may irritate skin.

*S   Geranium oil – essential oil; astringent; antiseptic; insect repellant; may irritate skin; frequent use may cause contact sensitization; see essential oils.

*S   Ginger oil – essential oil; antiseptic; may cause photosensitivity; frequent use may cause contact sensitization; see essential oils.

C   Ginseng – herb; demulcent; stimulant; may increase cell life; may cause vaginal bleeding.

X   Glutamic acid – non-essential amino acid; when used singly and out of balance with other amino acids, it is a source of hidden MSG; skin, eye, respiratory and digestive irritant; mutagen, may cause birth defects; harmful if absorbed through skin, swallowed or inhaled; suspected carcinogen; not adequately tested.

*C   Glycerin – derived from plant or animal fats and oils; see glycerol.

*C   Glycerine – derived from plant or animal fats and oils; see glycerol.

*C   Glycerol – may be derived from animal and vegetable fats and oils or produced synthetically from petroleum; nontoxic as used; drying to skin with repeated use; in concentrated form, may irritate eyes, skin and mucous membranes; mildly toxic by ingestion; chronic exposure may harm kidneys; safety claims not proven in diaper-rash, poison ivy, oak and sumac products; not adequately tested.

†CA   Glycerol monolaurate – synthetic; skin irritant; may cause contact dermatitis.

†CA   Glycerol monostearate – synthetic; eye irritant; may cause contact dermatitis.

†CA   Glyceryl laurate – synthetic; CIR says safe as used; see glyceryl monolaurate.

†CA   Glyceryl monolaurate – synthetic; skin irritant; may cause contact dermatitis; CIR says safe as used; see glyceryl oleate.

†CA   Glyceryl monooleate – synthetic; see glyceryl oleate.

†CA   Glyceryl monostearate – synthetic; eye irritant; see glyceryl oleate.

†CA   Glyceryl oleate – synthetic; eye and skin irritant; may cause contact dermatitis; a monoglyceride; made from hydrogenated oil; CIR panel says safe as used.

CA   Glyceryl PABA – synthetic; may cause photosensitivity, skin irritation.

X   Glyceryl ricinoleate – synthetic; insufficient data to support safety according to CIR panel; not adequately tested.

†CA   Glyceryl stearate – synthetic; CIR says safe as used; see glyceryl monostearate.

†CA   Glyceryl thioglycolate – synthetic; skin irritant in permanent solutions; potential sensitizer; CIR panel says safe if ≤15.4% as thiogly.

*C   Glycyl alcohol – see glycerol.

CA   Glycols – synthetic petroleum derivative; FDA says may cause adverse reactions; toxicity varies among different glycols; hazardous when used on large areas of the body; see butylene glycol, ethylene glycol, pentylene glycol, propylene glycol.

†CA   Glycol distearate – synthetic; may irritate eyes, skin and mucous membranes; may be contaminated with ethylene glycol; see ethylene glycol; CIR says safe as used.

†C   Glycolic acid – synthetic; see alpha hydroxy acids.

†C   Glycolic acid + ammonium glycolate – synthetic; see alpha hydroxy acids.

†C   Glycomer in crosslinked fatty acids alpha nutrium – synthetic; see alpha hydroxy acids.

CA   Glyoxylic acid – synthetic; corrosive; eye and skin
      irritant; sensitizer; mutagen in lab animals; on CIR
      high priority review list.
C1   Goldenseal extract – herb;natural antibiotic; immune
      system stimulant; aids digestion; healing to skin and
      mucous membranes; may increase blood pressure,
      stimulate uterus; avoid if pregnant or hypertensive;
      toxic in large amounts.
C1   Gotu kola – herb; anti-wrinkle; anti-aging properties;
      avoid if pregnant or lactating.
S   Grain alcohol – natural.
*C   Grapefruit seed extract – synthetic; derived from
      grapefruit seeds and pulp; one study showed
      contamination with benzethonium chloride in most
      of the samples tested and triclosan and methyl
      paraben in fewer of the samples, each of which
      showed antimicrobial activity; the sample without
      preservatives had no antimicrobial activity; this
      study concluded that antimicrobial activity was due
      to the chemical preservatives detected. However, a
      major supplier of grapefruit seed extract, states that
      their grapefruit seed extract products have been
      "proven clean" and effective by independent
      laboratory tests; see page 28.
C   Grapeseed oil   essential oil carrier; astringent; may
      be extracted with petrochemicals.
φXA   Green No. 3 – synthetic; carcinogen; see FD&C
      Green No. 3.
φC   Guaiazulene – plant derived; not adequately tested;
      CIR panel states insufficient data to support safety;
      see external use only.
φC   Guanine – plant, animal or synthetically derived; a
      constituent of DNA and RNA; skin, eye irritant, may
      be harmful if inhaled, engested; not adequately
      tested.
C   Guar gum – plant derived; possible eye, skin irritant;
      may be harmful if absorbed through skin, inhaled,

ingested; avoid long-term skin, inhalation exposure; not considered hazardous; not adequately tested.

XA   Guar hydroxypropyltrimonium chloride – synthetic; see quarternary ammonium compounds.

X   Hair dyes – synthetic; cause cancer, but do not require a warning on the label; increase risk of multiple myeloma, Hodgkin's disease, non-Hodgkin's lymphoma and possibly breast cancer; increase risk of bladder cancer by as much as 50%; greater risk with darker colors and permanent dyes.

CA   Hamamelis virginiana – plant derived; see witch hazel.

X   HC Blue No. 1 – synthetic; carcinogen, IARC Group 2B; CIR panel determined this ingredient to be unsafe.

†XA   HC Red No. 3 – synthetic; coal tar dye, used in hair dyes; mutagen; contains nitrosamines; IARC Group 3; not adequately tested; CIR says safe as used in hair dyes, but should not be used in products containing N-nitrosating agents.

*S   Helichrysum – essential oil; antioxidant; sunscreen; see essential oils.

*S   Helichrysum italicum – see helichrysum.

φCA   Henna – plant derived, but some hennas may also have synthetic colors; skin irritant; avoid use near eyes; limited to hair dyes; pure henna is safe; black or colored henna is not pure and may contain harmful chemicals .

C   Heliotrope oil – essential oil; skin, eye irritant; sensitizer; see essential oils.

X   Hexachlorophene – synthetic; extremely toxic; use prohibited unless physician prescribes; IARC Group 3.

†C   Hexadecanoic acid – synthetic; see palmitic acid.

†C   2,4-hexadienoic acid – synthetic; see sorbic acid.

†CA   Hexamethylenetetramine – synthetic; see methenamine.

C   Hexamidine diisethionate – synthetic; skin irritant; petroleum based; many petroleum products are carcinogens.

†XA   Hexylene glycol – synthetic; eye, skin, mucous membrane irritant; toxic if inhaled or ingested; hazardous if used on large areas of the body; CIR says safe as used.

†CA   HMTA – synthetic; see methenamine.

XA   Homosalate – synthetic; coal tar derivative; endocrine disrupter; may cause allergic reaction.

CA   Homomenthyl salicylate – synthetic; see salicylic acid.

C   Hops – herb; antimicrobial; antiaging; may cause dermatitis.

C   Horse chestnut – herb, anti-inflammatory, for sensitive skin, capillary fragility; avoid if kidney problems, pregnant or nursing; not for children; not to be used with blood-thinning drugs.

C1   Horsetail – herb; avoid if pregnant; excess may cause birth defects.

C   Humulus lupulus – see hops.

CA   Hyaluronic acid – see sodium hyaluronate.

C   Hydantoins – synthetic; skin irritant; has caused cancer in rats.

C   Hydrated silica – natural mineral; see silica.

X   Hydrazine – synthetic; skin and eye irritant; carcinogen, IARC Group 2B.

X   Hydrochlorofluorocarbon 22 – synthetic; propellant; respiratory irritant; may cause confusion, tremors; skin contact may cause defatting of the skin; sniffing fumes is hazardous, can cause death; IARC Group 3; depletes ozone; to be phased out in U.S. between 2010 and 2020; on CIR high priority review list.

X   Hydrochlorofluorocarbon 142B – synthetic; see hydrochlorofluorocarbon 22

C1   Hydrocotyle asiatica – see gotu kola.

X   Hydrofluorocarbon 134A – synthetic; propellant; skin and eye irritant; can cause frostbite; may cause loss of concentration, dizziness; high levels may cause cardiac arrhythmia, central nervous system disorders; in confined areas, may cause asphyxiation; on CIR high priority review list.

X Hydrofluorocarbon 152A – synthetic; propellant; eye, nose and throat irritant; may cause pulmonary irritation, lightheadedness, confusion, tremors; on CIR high priority review list.

*C Hydrogen peroxide – synthetic; toxic if inhaled or large amounts ingested; mutagen; skin irritant undiluted; 3% solution considered safe as antiseptic, gargle; not proven safe for poison ivy, poison oak, poison sumac; IARC Group 3.

CA Hydrogenated oils – synthetic; trans fats; absorbed directly into the bloodstream; interfere with prostaglandin activity in the body; essential fatty acids and fat soluble vitamins destroyed; consumption is associated with heart disease, breast and colon cancer, atherosclerosis, elevated cholesterol.

C Hydrogenated Polyisobutene – synthetic; petroleum derivative; penetrates skin rapidly; synthetic substitute for squalane; not adequately tested; on CIR high priority review list; see hydrogenated oils.

CA Hydrogenated vegetable oil – synthetic; trans fats; absorbed directly into the bloodstream; interfere with prostaglandin activity in the body; essential fatty acids and fat soluble vitamins destroyed; consumption is associated with heart disease, breast and colon cancer, atherosclerosis, elevated cholesterol.

C Hydrolyzed – process may involve use of an acid or enzyme which may be genetically modified; contains hidden MSG; see MSG.

C Hydrolyzed protein – synthetic; causes the formation of MSG or processed free glutamic acid; see MSG.

C Hydrolyzed whole wheat protein – synthetic; contains hidden MSG; see MSG.

XA Hydroquinol – synthetic; see hydroquinone.

†XA   Hydroquinone – synthetic; may cause severe skin damage; toxic if inhaled or ingested; ingesting less than 1 ounce may be fatal; has caused cancer in mice; IARC Group 3; CIR panel says safe at .1% concentrations or less for brief, "rinse-off" use only, NOT for non-drug leave-on products; see external use only; banned in Europe.

CA   Hydroxy citronellal – synthetic; skin and eye irritant; may cause psoriasis, contact dermatitis; harmful if swallowed.

X   p-hydroxyanisole – synthetic; CIR panel determined this ingredient to be unsafe.

C   Hydroxybenzoic acids – synthetic; see salicylic acid.

†C   Hydroxycaprylic acid – synthetic; see alpha hydroxy acids.

CA   Hydroxycitronella – synthetic; see hydroxy citronellal.

CA   Hydroxycoumarins – synthetic; skin irritant; may cause photosensitivity; coumarin is a carcinogen and banned in food.

C   Hydroxyethyl Acrylate/Sodium Acryloyldimethyl Taurate Copolymer – synthetic; considered low hazard and not a risk to the environment, but in case of waste or accidental spill, it is to be disposed of in a sealed container in a landfill, not in the water system.

CA   2-hydroxyethylamine – synthetic; see ethanolamine.

†CA   Hydroxyethylcellulose – synthetic; may cause skin, eye, respiratory irritation; not adequately tested; CIR says safe as used.

C   2-hydroxy-4-methoxybenzophenone – synthetic; can cause serious contact dermatitis.

C   Hydroxymethylcellulose – synthetic; see carboxymethyl cellulose.

CA   2-hydroxypropyl amine – synthetic; see monoisopropanolamine.

C   Hydroxypropyl aminobenzoate – synthetic; may cause formation of carcinogens in products containing nitrogen compounds.

†CA   <u>Hydroxypropyl cellulose</u> – synthetic; slight skin and eye irritant; overexposure may cause harm if inhaled, ingested or absorbed through skin; no long term safety studies; CIR says safe as used; see cellulose gum.

C   <u>Hydroxypropyl guar</u> – plant derived; no known toxicity; see guar gum.

†CA   <u>Hydroxy propylmethyl cellulose</u> – synthetic; skin and eye irritant; CIR says safe as used; see cellulose gum.

C1   <u>Hypericum perforatum</u> – herb; essential oil: anti-inflammatory; antibiotic; astringent; skin irritant; causes photosensitivity; avoid if pregnant.

C1   <u>Hypericum perforatum extract</u> – herb; essential oil: anti-inflammatory; antibiotic; astringent; skin irritant; causes photosensitivity; avoid if pregnant; insufficient data to support safety according to CIR panel.

C1   <u>Hypericum perforatum oil</u> – herb; essential oil: anti-inflammatory; antibiotic; astringent; skin irritant; causes photosensitivity; avoid if pregnant; insufficient data to support safety according to CIR panel.

*C1   <u>Hyssop oil</u> – essential oil; astringent; antiseptic; contains pinocamphone which may be toxic; avoid if pregnant, epileptic or high blood pressure; see essential oils.

*C   <u>Hyssopus officinalis</u> – see hyssop oil.

†C   <u>Imidazolidinyl urea</u> – synthetic; preservative; strong irritant; causes contact deramtitis; may contain formaldehyde; see formaldehyde; CIR says safe as used.

C   <u>Indian Cress</u> – herb, antibacterial, antifungal; may have anti-cancer effects; safety data not found.

*S   <u>Inositol</u> – a B vitamin; see nutrient additives.

CA   <u>Iodine</u> – naturally occuring element; skin and eye irritant; may cause asthma or anaphylactic shock in susceptible individuals.

C   <u>Irish moss</u> – plant derived; see carrageenan.

φC   Iron oxides – natural or synthetic; slight skin, eye and respiratory irritant; harmful if absorbed through skin; may cause siderosis from occupational exposure; may contain contaminants of lead, arsenic, cadmium, beryllium; see micronized minerals.

†C   Isobutane – petroleum derivative; propellant; flammable; neurotoxin; CIR says safe as used.

C   Isoceteth-n – synthetic; may contain toxic byproducts; see ethoxylated alcohols.

CA   Isocetyl laurate – synthetic; see isocetyl stearate.

CA   Isocetyl stearate – synthetic; mild skin, eye, respiratory irritant; may cause acne; not adequately tested.

X   Isoeugenol – synthetic; strong skin irritant; mutagen; toxic if swallowed.

C   Isolaureth-n – synthetic; may contain toxic byproducts; see ethoxylated alcohols.

†C   Isopentane – synthetic; petroleum derivative; skin irritant; flammable; narcotic in large amounts; CIR says safe as used.

†CA   Isopropanolamine – synthetic; CIR panel says safe but not in products with N-nitrosating agents; see monoisopropanloamine.

C   4-isopropyl-dibenzoylmethane – synthetic; can cause contact dermatitis.

CA   Isopropyl-hydroxypalmityl-ether – synthetic; may cause allergic reactions.

†C   Isopropyl isostearate – synthetic; may cause acne; mild skin irritant; not adequately tested; CIR says safe as used.

†XA   Isopropyl myristate – synthetic; may cause acne, irritate skin; may increase absorption of toxic/carcinogenic contaminants by more than 200 times; CIR says safe as used.

†CA   Isopropyl palmitate – synthetic; may irritate skin, cause acne; not aequately tested; CIR says safe as used.

C   Isopsoralen – synthetic; causes phototoxicity; IARC Group 3.

†C   Isostearamide DEA – synthetic; may cause formation of carcinogens in products containing nitrogen compounds; CIR panel says safe for use in rinse-off products, OK for leave-on products that limit the release of ethanolamines to 5%, but a maximum concentration of 40%, not to be used in products where N-nitroso compounds may form; see DEA.

†C   Isostearamide MEA – synthetic; see isostearamide DEA.

C   Isosteareth -20 – synthetic; may contain toxic byproducts; see ethoxylated alcohols.

C   Isosteareth -n – synthetic; may contain toxic byproducts; see ethoxylated alcohols.

†C   Isostearic acid – synthetic; skin, eye and mucous membrane irritant; potential sensitizer; not adequately tested; CIR says safe as used.

†C   Isostearyl neopentanoate – synthetic; may cause acne; not adequately tested; CIR says safe as used.

CA   Isothiazolinones – synthetic; preservative; may irritate skin, cause allergic reaction, mostly in those with nickel allergies; mutagen.

S   Ispaghul extract – herb; see plantago.

C1A   Ivy extract – plant extract; skin irritant; may cause dermatitis; toxic if taken internally; not recommended for children or during pregnancy.

C1   Jasmine – see essential oils.

C1   Jasmine absolute – essential oil; antiseptic; anti-inflammatory; antibacterial; not for use during first 8 months of pregnancy; facilitates labor; see essential oils.

C1   Jasminum officinale – see jasmine absolute.

†SA   Jojoba oil – plant derived; healing to skin, natural sunscreen if cold pressed; heat pressed or solvent extracted is highly refined and loses healing properties; CIR says safe as used.

*C1   Juniper oil – essential oil; antibacterial; anti-inflammatory; astringent; detoxifier; avoid if kidney problems and during pregnancy; see essential oils.

*C1   Juniperus communis – see juniper oil.

†C   Kaolin clay – natural clay; contains crystalline silica, aluminum silicates; skin and eye irritant; may cause gastrointestinal distress if ingested; long term exposure of dust may cause cancer; no known toxicity for the skin; CIR says safe as used.

CA   Kathon CG – synthetic; sensitizer; skin and eye irritant; low toxicity; see methylchloroisothiazolinone and methylisothiazolinone.

S   Keratin protein – a component of skin, nails and hair; animal derived.

X   Kohl – made with antimony or soot; causes lead poisoning.

S   Kukui nut oil – carrier oil; healing properties.

†C   Lactic acid – naturally derived from milk or synthetically produced; see alpha hydroxy acids.

C   Lacto-ceramide – see ceramide 3.

†C   L-alpha hydroxy acid – see alpha hydroxy acids.

†CA   Lanolin – derived from sheep's wool; skin irritant; sensitizer; may cause cheilitis; safety and effectiveness not shown for poison oak, ivy and sumac products; may be contaminated with carcinogenic and neurotoxic pesticides which may be absorbed through the skin into the bloodstream; should be avoided by nursing mothers, infants and children; highly refined and purified lanolin is free of contaminants, allergens and irritants and is safe for all, including nursing mothers and infants; CIR says safe as used.

CA   Lanolin alcohol – derived from sheep's wool; may cause acne; less irritating than lanolin; may be contaminated with carcinogenic and neurotoxic pesticides; should be avoided by nursing mothers and infants and children; see lanolin.

†CA   Lanolin oil – derived from sheep's wool; may be less irritating to skin than lanolin; may be contaminated with carcinogenic and neurotoxic pesticides; should

be avoided by nursing mothers and infants and children; see lanolin.

†C   **Lauramide DEA** – synthetic detergent; may cause formation of carcinogens in products containing nitrogen compounds; CIR panel says safe in products that do not contain nitrosating agents; see DEA.

CA   **Lauramidopropyl dimethylamine** – synthetic; skin, mucous membrane irritant.

*C   **Laurel oil** – essential oil; frequent use may cause contact sensitization; possible skin irritant; use cautiously or avoid if pregnant; see bay oil, essential oils.

†C   **Laureth-1, -23** – synthetic; may contain toxic byproducts; CIR says safe as used for -4, -23;see ethoxylated alcohols.

*C1   **Laurus nobilis** – essential oil; see laurel oil.

†C   **Lauroyl sarcosine** – derived from sea urchins, starfish, caffeine; skin irritant; penetration enhancer; CIR panel says safe in "rinse-off" products, safe at ≤5% concentrations in "leave-on" products, insufficient data to determine safety in products which might be inhaled, may cause formation of carcinogens in products containing nitrogen compounds.

C   **Lauryl alcohol** – synthetic; may cause acne, slight irritant to skin and eyes; not adequately tested for long-term exposure.

CA   **Laurylpyridinium Chloride** – synthetic; see quaternary ammonium compounds; on CIR high priority review list.

*C1   **Lavandin** – essential oil; antiseptic; anti-inflammatory; avoid if pregnant; use cautiously or avoid if epileptic; do not use for burns; not the same as lavender oil; see essential oils.

*C1   **Lavandula Delphinensis** – see lavandin.

*C1   **Lavandula Fragrans** – see lavandin.

*S   **Lavandula officinalis** – see lavender oil.

*S   Lavender oil – essential oil; antiseptic; anti-inflammatory; may cause photosensitivity; skin irritant; see essential oils.

*S   Lavendula officinalis – see lavender oil.

ϕX   Lead acetate – synthetic; absorption through skin may cause lead poisoning; carcinogen, IARC Group 2A; reproductive toxin; limited to hair dyes; banned in Europe.

†C   Lecithin – derived from plant or animal sources; CIR says safe in "rinse-off" products, safe in "leave-on" products up to 15% concentration, insufficient data to determine safety where ingredients might be inhaled, may cause formation of carcinogens in products containing nitrogen compounds.

*S   Lemon – see lemon juice.

*C1   Lemon balm – see melissa oil.

*C1   Lemon balm oil – see melissa oil.

*C1   Lemon essence – see lemon oil.

*C1   Lemon extract – see lemon oil.

*S   Lemon juice – may cause photosensitivity; may irritate the skin.

*C1   Lemon oil – essential oil from lemon peel; may cause phototoxicity; antiseptic; antibacterial; anti-aging properties; may cause contact dermatitis; avoid if pregnant; see essential oils.

*S   Lemon peel

*C1   Lemon peel oil – see lemon oil.

*C1   Lemongrass oil – essential oil; skin irritant; antibacterial; antifungal; insect repellant; mildly toxic if swallow large amounts; topical safety unknown; use small amounts; avoid with glaucoma; caution with sensitive or damaged skin and prostatic hyperplasia; avoid with children; avoid if pregnant.

S   Lichen – botanical; antimicrobial, antibiotic; no known toxicity

*C1   Lime essence – see lime oil.

*S   Lime juice – see lemon juice.

*C1   Lime oil – essential oil; antiseptic; anti-bacterial; anti-viral; phototoxic; use in very low concentrations; avoid if pregnant; see essential oils.

C   d-limonene – synthetic; sensitizer; skin and eye irritant; inadequate evidence of carcinogenity; teratogen; neurotoxin; IARC Group 3.

C   Linalol – see linalool.

C   Linalool – essential oil; skin irritant.

†C   Lineoleamide DEA – synthetic; can cause formation of carcinogens in products containing nitrogen compounds; CIR panel says safe, but should not be used in products with nitrosating agents; see DEA.

C   Linoleamidopropyl ethydimonium ethosulfate – synthetic; may cause formation of carcinogens in products containing nitrogen compounds; skin and mucous membrane irritant; contains ammonium salts, see ammonia.

SA   Linseed oil – plant extract: may cause acne.

C   Liposomes – natural or synthetic; spherical vesicles derived from cholesterol and phosolipids that act as carriers to deliver enzymes, drugs, vaccines into the body; used in cosmetics for moisturizing, delivering cosmetic ingredients to the horny layer of the skin; liposomal delivery systems are experimental; safety data not available.

†C   Magnesium aluminum silicate – refined, purified smectite clay; bentonite; naturally occuring mineral; contains a small amount of crystalline silica <10%; skin, eye, respiratory irritant; ingesting large quantities causes systemic alkalosis; adverse effects primarily due to occupational exposure and inhalation of the dust; hydrated magnesium aluminum silicate long fibers IARC Group 2B, short fibers Group 3; no adverse effects when applied to skin; CIR says safe as used.

X   Magnesium fluoride – synthetic; toxic; eye, skin irritant; harmful if ingested, inhaled; not adequately tested; IARC Group 3; see fluoride.

X   Magnesium fluorosilicate – synthetic; toxic; severe skin irritant; harmful if ingested, inhaled; long term overexposure through inhalation or ingestion could be fatal; skin absorption can cause fluorosis, with symptoms like brittle bones, weight loss, anemia, stiff joints, weakness, internal bleeding; IARC Group 3; see fluoride.

C   Magnesium laureth sulfate – synthetic; may contain toxic byproducts; contains ammonium salts; see ammonia, ethoxylated alcohols.

C   Magnesium oleth sulfate – synthetic; may contain toxic byproducts; contains ammonium salts; see ammonia, ethoxylated alcohols.

CA   Maize oil – may be genetically modified; see corn oil.

†C   Malic acid – fruit extract; CIR panel says safe as pH adjuster only, insufficient data to determine safety for any other use; see alpha hydroxy acids; do not use on children.

S   Mallow – herb; antiallergenic; anti-inflammatory; for sensitive skin.

C   Maltitol – sugar alcohol; causes gastrointestinal distress when ingested in large amounts; produced from hydrogenated maltose; may be corn or wheat based; on CIR high priority review list.

S   Malva sylvestris – herb; see mallow.

*S   Mandarin oil – essential oil; antiseptic; gentle; may be used for children and during pregnancy; causes photosensitivity; see essential oils.

φC   Manganese violet – synthetic; eye irritant; toxic if inhaled; approved for use around the eyes; presumed safe; not adequately tested; contains ammonium and phosphates.

S   Marigold – herb; soothes inflammation; may cause dermatitis.

C   Marigold oil – essential oil; may cause photosensitivity; see marigold, oils.

*C1 Marjoram oil – essential oil; antiseptic; anti-bacterial; use cautiously or avoid if pregnant; see essential oils.

S Marshmallow – herb; may heal eczema, dermatitis.

C1A Matricaria chamomilla – see chamomile.

CA MEA – synthetic; see monoethanolamine.

C Meadowfoam seed oil – plant derived; stable moisturizing oil from the seed of the meadowfoam herb; not adequately tested.

C1 Meadowsweet oil – essential oil; avoid if aspirin sensitive, pregnant; do not give to children with chicken-pox, colds, flu.

*S Melaleuca alternifolia – essential oil; antiseptic; anti-bacterial; anti-fungal; anti-viral; frequent use may cause contact sensitization; see essential oils.

S Melaleuca ericifolia – essential oil; see rosalina.

*C1 Melaleuca leucadendron – essential oil; see cajaput oil.

*S Melaleuca quinquenervia – essential oil; see melaleuca alternifolia.

*S Melaleuca viridiflora – essential oil; see melaleuca alternifolia.

*C1 Melissa balm oil – see melissa oil.

*C1 Melissa oil – essential oil; insect repellant; antibacterial; calming; may interfere with thyroid hormones; often distilled with other oils; may not be pure; external use only; caution if pregnant; see essential oils.

*C1 Melissa officinalis – see melissa oil.

*C1 Mentha piperita – essential oil; see peppermint oil.

*C1 Mentha spicata – essential oil; see spearmint oil.

C Menthol – can be plant derived or synthetic; eye irritant; moderately toxic if swallowed in large amounts; local anesthetic; may cause changes in the mucous membranes if used for long periods in concentrations greater than 3%; FDA says not shown safe and effective in over-the-counter products.

X   Mercuric ammonium chloride – synthetic; poison; mercury compounds are prohibited except as preservatives in eye cosmetics; see ammonia.

X   Mercuric chloride – synthetic; poison; mercury compounds are prohibited except as preservatives in eye cosmetics.

X   Mercuric chloride ammoniated – synthetic; toxic; skin irritant; mercury compounds are prohibited except as preservatives in eye cosmetics; see ammonia.

XA   Methanal – synthetic; see formaldehyde.

†XA   Methaninie – synthetic; see quaternium 15.

†XA   Methenamine – synthetic; CIR says safe if $\leq$16%, but NOT in aerosol products; see quaternium 15.

X   Methanol – synthetic solvent; see methyl alcohol.

X   Methenammonium chloride – synthetic; see ammonia.

X   Methoxsalen – synthetic; phototoxic chemical, causes photosensitivity, may damage DNA and cause mutations, tumors or neoplasms; carcinogen, IARC Group 1.

X   2-methoxyaniline – synthetic; irritant; harmful if absorbed through skin, inhaled, ingested; sensitizer; carcinogen; IARC Group 2B.

C   4-methoxyaniline – synthetic; harmful if absorbed through skin or inhaled; may cause contact dermatitis; sensitizer; IARC Group 3.

X   4-methoxy-3-phenylenediamine – synthetic; carcinogen; CIR says unsafe for use in cosmetics.

X   4-methoxy-m-phenylenediamine – synthetic; carcinogen; CIR panel determined this ingredient to be unsafe.

X   4-methoxy-m-phenylenediamine HCl – synthetic; CIR panel determined this ingredient to be unsafe.

X   4-methoxy-m-phenylenediamine sulfate – synthetic; CIR panel determined this ingredient to be unsafe; contains ammonium salts, see ammonia.

X   5-methoxypsoralen – synthetic; phototoxic chemical, may damage DNA and cause mutations, tumors or neoplasms; probable carcinogen; IARC Group 2A; banned in Europe.

X   8-methoxypsoralen – synthetic; see methoxsalen; banned in Europe.

†X   Methyl alcohol – synthetic; mutagen; neurotoxin; skin and eye irritant; mild toxicity if inhaled; poison if swallowed; may cause blindness; CIR says safe as used to denature alcohol used in cosmetic products.

XA   3-Methylamino-4-Nitrophenoxyethanol – synthetic; used in hair dyes; skin irritant; has caused reduced blood oxygen, restlessness, convulsions; on CIR high priority review list.

C   Methyl-alpha-d-glycopyranoside – synthetic; skin irritant.

C   Methyl benzoate – synthetic; associated with numerous health issues; has caused skin irritation in lab animals; toxic if ingested.

C   Methyl ester – synthetic; see methyl benzoate.

C   Methyl gluceth – synthetic; may contain toxic byproducts; see ethoxylated alcohols.

C   Methyl glucose sesquistearate – synthetic; skin irritant; not adequately tested.

C   Methyl glucoside – synthetic; skin and eye irritant; may be harmful if inhaled or ingested; not adequately tested.

CA   3-methyl isothiazolin – synthetic; can cause contact allergies.

CA   3-methyl isothiazolinone – synthetic; see isothiazolinones.

XA   Methyl methacrylate – synthetic; glue used with artificial nail products; skin, eye and nail irritant; absorbed through skin, lungs, gastrointestinal tract; high level exposure may cause behavioral, neurochemical, bone marrow, brain kidney and liver changes; low level exposure can affect the liver; posssible heart and neurotoxic effects in occupationally exposed; developmental effects to fetus have occurred in lab animals; no reproductive studies have been performed; flammable; banned in Canada; IARC Group 3; not adequately tested.

†C   Methyl oleate – synthetic; may cause acne; skin irritant; not adequately tested.

C   Methyl salicylate – synthetic; eye, skin and mucous membrane irritant; poison if swallowed; swallowing causes nausea, vomiting, shortness of breath; highly absorbable through skin; ingestion of small amounts has caused death; as of February 2000, CIR panel tentatively concluded this is safe when formulated to avoid irritation, and when formulated to avoid increasing sun sensitivity, if sun sensitivity is expected, directions should include use of sun protection.

†*S   Methylcellulose – synthetic; skin and eye irritant; CIR says safe as used.

†CA   Methylchloroisothiazolinone – synthetic; preservative; strong allergen; CIR panel says safe with qualifications.

†CA   Methyldibromo glutaronitrile – synthetic; preservative; skin irritant; skin absorbs readily; CIR panel says safe in "rinse-off" products, and up to .025% in "leave-on" products

†CA   Methylisothiazolinone – synthetic preservative; strong allergen; CIR panel says safe with qualifications.

CA   2-methyl-4-isothiazolin-3-one – synthetic; can cause allergies, contact dermatitis.

C   6-methylquinophthalone – synthetic; can cause dermatitis.

†CA   Methylparaben – synthetic preservative; mutagen; toxic if swallowed; associated with numerous of health problems, including contact dermatitis and asthma; endocrine disrupter; strong allergen: CIR says safe as used, but CIR is re-evaluating safety.

CA   Methyl-p-hydroxybenzoate – synthetic; see methylparaben.

CA   Methyl/propyl paraben – synthetic; see methylparaben, propyl paraben.

X 7-methylpyrido[3,4-c]psoralen – synthetic; phototoxic chemical, may damage DNA and cause mutations, tumors or neoplasms.

†X Methylene chloride – synthetic; carcinogen, IARC Group 2B; mutagen; may damage central nervous system, kidneys and liver; skin and eye irritant; inhalation causes headaches, tremors, nervousness, insomnia; CIR says safe for brief discontinuous use.

†C Mexenone – synthetic; see benzophenone.

φC Mica – minerals; inhalation may damage lungs; nontoxic to skin; considered safe; safety data not available.

CA Microcrystalline wax – petroleum derivative, from distillation of crude oil; prolonged exposure may irritate skin; not adequately tested.

X Micronized minerals – minerals; can be absorbed into the cell and damage the DNA; can cross the blood brain barrier; particles <1 micron are pathogenic and cause disease; toxic; not adequately tested.

X Micronized titanium dioxide – minerals; see micronized minerals.

X Micronized zinc dioxide – minerals; see micronized minerals.

X Mineral oil – petroleum derivative; phototoxin; eye and skin irritant; may cause acne, birth defects; clogs pores; embryotoxic, teratogenic to birds; potential carcinogen; may contain carcinogenic contaminants; IARC Group 1 for untreated and mildly treated mineral oils; IARC Group 3 for highly refined mineral oils.

†C Mink oil – synthetic; penetration enhancer; may contain harmful impurities; CIR Expert Panel says safe as used.

CA MIPA – synthetic; see monoisopropanolamine.

†C mixed fruit acid – see alpha hydroxy acids.

XA MMA – synthetic; see methyl methacrylate.

C MMP inhibitors – MMP's are extracellular proteolytic enzymes that appear to be involved with various pathological processes, including inflammation, arthritis and cancer. MMP inhibitors are considered a promising therapy for treatment of tumors, arthritis and wound healing, but have shown little therapeutic effect; used in cosmetics to reduce activity of enzymes that cause aging; safety data not available; toxological properties not fully investigated.

C   Modulan – synthetic; skin irritant; has caused tissue changes and skin irritation in lab animals.

C   Monoazoanilies – synthetic; may cause acne.

†CA   Monoethanolamine – synthetic; toxic if absorbed through skin; severe irritant to skin, eyes, respiratory and digestive tracts; may cause swelling, redness, tissue damage; ongoing overexposure may cause kidney, liver damage; not studied for carcinogenic effects; CIR panel says safe up to 5% concentration in "rinse-off" products only; see ethanolamine.

CA   Monoethanolamine lauryl sulfate – synthetic; may cause formation of carcinogens in products containing nitrogen compounds; contains ammonium salts; see ammonia, monoethanolamine.

CA   Monoethanolamine sulfite – synthetic; skin irritant; contains ammonium salts; see ammonia, monoethanolamine.

CA   Monoisopropanolamine – synthetic; skin and eye irritant; may cause formation of carcinogens in products containing nitrogen compounds.

CA   Monophenyl ether – synthetic; can cause contact dermatitis, allergic reactions.

CA   Monotertiary butyl hydroquinone – synthetic; can cause contact dermatitis, allergic reactions.

*C   Mountain savory – essential oil; severe skin and mucous membrane irritant; never use undiluted; exercise extreme caution; avoid if pregnant.

*XA   MSG – synthetic or through bacterial fermentation, bacteria are genetically modified; may cause headaches, itching, nausea, brain, nervous system, reproductive disorders, high blood pressure;

109

pregnant, lactating mothers, infants, children women of child-bearing age and people with affective disorders should avoid; allergic reactions common; may be hidden in cosmetics, hair conditioners, shampoos, soaps, infant formula, low fat milk, candy, chewing gum, drinks, processed foods, over-the-counter and prescription medications, especially children's, binders and fillers for nutritional supplements, prescription and non-prescription drugs, IV fluids given in hospitals, chicken pox vaccine; it is being sprayed on some growing fruits and vegetables, primarily as a pesticide that enhances growth and increases yield and product size.

CA   Musk – animal derived; may cause allergic reactions; eye, skin, respiratory irritant; overexposure may cause dizziness, breathing difficulty.

*CA   Musk ambrette – synthetic; petroleum derivative; causes photosensitivity; skin irritant; may damage myelin nerve coverings; IARC Group 3; banned in Europe.

CA   Musk moskene – synthetic; may cause skin hyperpigmentation, dermatitis; skin irritant.

C   Mustard oil – essential oil; burns the skin if used improperly; avoid if allergies or nervous conditions.

CA   Myristamidopropyl dimethylamine – synthetic; skin irritant; potentially toxic.

C   Myristates –synthetic; may cause acne; may be toxic.

†CA   Myristic acid – synthetic; skin irritant; mutagen; CIR says safe as used.

C   Myristica fragrans – essential oil; see nutmeg oil.

†CA   Myristyl alcohol – synthetic; skin irritant; may cause acne; not adequately tested; CIR says safe as used.

†CA   Myristyl lactate – synthetic; sensitizer; penetration enhancer; may cause acne; CIR says safe with many qualifications, including brief use followed by thorough rinsing; used in lip pencils, lip gloss,

lipstick and eye make-up, which are all unsafe uses; see alpha hydroxy acids.

†C   Myristyl myristate – synthetic; may cause acne; mild skin and eye irritant; nontoxic in animal studies; not adequately tested; CIR says safe as used.

C   Myristyl propionate – synthetic; may cause acne; not evaluated by CIR; not adequately tested.

*C1   Myrrh – see myrrh oil.

*C1   Myrrh oil – essential oil; antiseptic; antifungal; immune stimulant; circulatory stimulant; uterine stimulant; avoid if pregnant or lactating; see essential oils.

*C1   Myrtle – essential oil; astringent; anti-bacterial; anti-inflammatory; avoid if pregnant; see essential oils.

C1   Myrtus communis – see myrtle.

†C   NaPCA – synthetic; may cause the formation of carcinogenic nitrosamines if product contains nitrogen compounds; otherwise CIR considers safe.

CA   Naphtha – synthetic; petroleum or coal tar derivative; skin irritant; may cause dry skin, difficulty breathing, dizziness.

XA   Naphthalene – synthetic; petroleum or coal tar derivative; skin and eye irritant; poison; potential carcinogen, IARC 2B; neurotoxin.

XA   Naphthol – synthetic; coal tar derivative; skin and eye irritant; poison; see coal tar derivatives.

†XA   1-naphthol – synthetic; coal tar derivative; used in hair dyes; severe irritant to eyes and skin; if absorbed through skin may cause liver damage, acute hemolytic anemia, severe nephritis; may cause convulsions; CIR says safe as used.

*S   Nardostachys jatamansi – essential oil; see spikenard.

C   Natural essence oils – see natural oils.

C   Natural oils – if cold pressed, contain substances beneficial for the skin; if solvent extracted or hot pressed, they are highly refined and most beneficial substances are destroyed, may contain contaminants; see specific oil.

CA Natural fragrance – potential sensitizer; may cause allergic dermatitis.

C Nayad – natural; potent yeast extract; source of hidden MSG; not adequately tested; no one knows how it works in the skin.

C n-butyl benzoate – synthetic; skin irritant in rabbits.

†CA N-cocamidoprpyl-N,N-dimethlglycine hydroxide inner salt – synthetic; see cocamidopropyl betaine.

S Neem – plant derived; many healing properties

XA Neomycin – synthetic; antibacterial; skin irritant; may cause contact dermatitis; toxic to kidneys; may affect hearing; has caused resistant strains of staphylococcus bacteria to develop.

C Neopentyl glycol dicaprylate/dicaprate – synthetic; diester of caprylic and capric acids and neopentyl glycol; neopentyl glycol is derived from propylene glycol, a petrochemical; lubricates and softens the skin; safety data not available; not adequately tested; no known toxicity; not evaluated by CIR.

*S Neroli oil – essential oil; antiseptic; anti-bacterial; anti-viral; see essential oils.

C Nettle – herb; healing properties; anti-aging; may irritate skin, interact with certain drugs; may not be safe to use if pregnant.

S Niacin – see vitamin B3.

XA Nickel – metal; skin irritant; may cause contact dermatitis, asthma, depression, kidney and brain damage; carcinogen, IARC Group 2B (metallic nickel); mutagen.

XA Nickel sulfate – synthetic; may cause contace dermatitis; skin irritant; may cause depression, kidney and brain damage; carcinogen, IARC Group 1 (nickel compounds); contains ammonium salts, see ammonia.

X Nicomethanol hydrofluoride – synthetic; toxic; see fluoride; not adequately tested.

C Niobe oil – synthetic; see methyl benzoate.

X Nitrilotriacetic acid – synthetic; irritant; possible carcinogen, IARC Group 2B.

X   o-nitro-p-aminophenol – synthetic; EPA classifies as carcinogen; banned in Europe.

X   Nitrobenzene – synthetic; toxic if inhaled, ingested or absorbed through the skin; skin absorbs rapidly; poison; possible carcinogen, IARC Group 2B.

†X   4-nitro-o-phenylenediamine – synthetic; mutagen, may cause genetic damage; not adequately tested.

X   2-nitrophenylenediamine – synthetic; mutagen, may cause genetic damage.

X   2-nitro-4-phenylenediamine – synthetic; IARC Group 3, mutagen, may cause genetic damage.

X   2-nitropropane – synthetic; possible carcinogen, IARC Group 2B.

X   Nitrosamines – formed during the manufacturing process when an amine, such as MEA, DEA or TEA, combines with a formaldehyde releasing preservative; absorb through skin readily; levels may increase over time after product is opened; carcinogens; mutagens; contains ammonium salts, see ammonia.

X   n-nitroso compounds – carcinogenic cosmetic contaminant; IARC Group 2A; contains ammonium salts, see ammonia.

X   n-nitroso-n-methylalkylamines – carcinogenic contaminant; IARC Group 2A; contains ammonium salts, see ammonia.

X   n-nitroso-n-methyltetradecyl amine – carcinogenic contaminant; IARC Group 2A; contains ammonium salts, see ammonia.

X   n-nitrosoalkanolamines – carcinogen; IARC Group 2A; contains ammonium salts, see ammonia.

X   n-nitrosobis(2-hydroxypropyl)amine – synthetic; carcinogen (induced pancreatic tumors in hamsters in NCI study); contains ammonium salts, see ammonia.

X   n-nitrosodiethanolamine – carcinogenic cosmetic contaminant; IARC Group 2B; easily absorbed through skin; contains ammonium salts, see ammonia.

X   <u>n-nitrosodimethylamine</u> – carcinogenic cosmetic contaminant, IARC Group 2A; contains ammonium salts, see ammonia.

X   <u>n-nitrosomorpholine</u> – carcinogenic cosmetic contaminant, IARC Group 2B; contains ammonium salts, see ammonia.

X   <u>Nonylphenol</u> – synthetic; toxic if skin contact and if swallowed; toxic to endocrine system; not adequately tested.

X   <u>4-NOPD</u> – synthetic; mutagen, may cause genetic damage; not adequately tested.

CA   <u>Novocain</u> – synthetic; skin irritant; may cause swelling, anxiety, asthma; respiratory arrest.

†X   <u>N-phenyl-p-phenylenediamine</u> – synthetic; used in hair dyes; toxic; may cause severe dermatitis, hives, swelling around the eyes, tearing, blindness; excessive use of hair dyes may cause skin sensitization, liver damage; may cause gastritis, high blood pressure, asthma, tremors, vertigo, convulsions, coma: CIR say safe at $\leq 1.7\%$ as a free base.

C   <u>n-propyl benzoate</u> – synthetic; associated with many health issues; causes inflammation in rabbits.

C   <u>n-propylamines</u> – synthetic; strong skin irritant; hazardous.

*C1   <u>Nutmeg oil</u> – essential oil; antiseptic; anti-inflammatory; supports adrenal glands; not recommended to use undiluted; caution if pregnant; see essential oils.

C   <u>Nutrient additives</u> – nutrients added to mostly refined and processed foods giving a false sense of nutritional value and can lead to nutritional imbalances; chemicals used in preparing nutrients added are not listed on the label.

CA   <u>Oak moss</u> – plant derived; skin irritant; sensitizer; mucous membrane irritant; avoid if pregnant, epilepsy.

†X   <u>o-aminophenol</u> – synthetic; used in hair dyes; eye irritant, skin sensitizer; may cause contact dermatitis,

restlessness, convulsions; inhalation may cause methemoglobinemia, bronchial asthma; mutagenic; CIR says safe as used.

SA   1-octadecanol – synthetic; eye, skin, respiratory irritant; see stearyl alcohol.

SA   Octadecyl alcohol – synthetic; see stearyl alcohol.

CA   Octhilinone – synthetic; see Kathon CG.

X   Octocrylene – synthetic; may be derived from coal tar; see phenol.

X   Octyl dimethyl PABA – synthetic; may cause formation of nitrosamines; endocrine disrupter; shown to increase growth of cancer cells.

X A   Octyl methoxycinnamate – synthetic; skin, eye irritant; killed mouse skin cells in 2000 study; endocrine disrupter; shown to increase growth of cancer cells; penetration enhancer.

†C   Octyl palmitate – synthetic; may cause acne; not adequately tested; CIR says safe as used; safety determined based upon data for a related chemical.

C   Octyl salicylate – synthetic; see salicylic acid.

†C   Octyl stearate – synthetic; may cause acne; not adequately tested; CIR says safe as used; safety determined based upon data for a related chemical.

X A   Octylacrylamide/acrylates/butylaminoethyl methacrylate copolymer – synthetic; causes allergic reactions if inhaled, eye, skin, respiratory, digestive irritant; can cause permanent eye, nervous system damage, liver damage; may contain hydroquinone benzoyl peroxide; see hydroquinone and benzoyle peroxide.

X A   Octylacrylamide/acrylates/butylaminoethyl methacrylate polymer – synthetic; causes allergic reactions if inhaled; may contain hydroquinone benzoyl peroxide; see hydroquinone and benzoyle peroxide.

C   Octyoxynol-n – synthetic; may contain toxic byproducts.

C   Oils – must be cold pressed to preserve any healing and beneficial properties; heat pressed or solvent-extracted oils are highly refined and have lost healing and beneficial properties; may contain contaminants from processing; see specific oil.

†SA   Oil of jojoba – plant derived; see jojoba oil, oils.

S   Oil of kuawa – plant derived; oil of guava; many healing properties; see oils.

S   Oil of kukui – plant derived; candlenut oil; carrier oil mixed with essential oils; see oils.

*Cl   Oil of lemongrass – essential oil; skin irritant; insect repellant; anti-fungal; antibacterial; see lemongrass oil, essential oils.

S   Oil of lilikoi – plant derived; passion fruit oil; see oils.

S   Oil of manako – plant derived; mango oil; see oils.

SA   Oil of mikana – plant derived; papaya oil; see oils.

X   Oil of mirbane – synthetic; see nitrobenzene; see oils.

*Cl   Oil of myrrh – essential oil; see myrrh oil, essential oils.

*S   Oil of orange – see orange oil; essential oils.

S   Oil of orchid – plant derived; healing properties; see oils.

S   Oil of plumeria – essential oil from tropical flower.

C   Oil of purcellin – synthetic; skin irritant.

S   Oil of Taro – oil of Polynesian root vegetable.

†S   Oil of wheat germ – natural.

*C   Oil of wintergreen – synthetic; see methyl salicylate.

†CA   Oleamide DEA – synthetic; may cause formation of carcinogens in products containing nitrogen compounds; mucous membrane and skin irritant; CIR panel says safe in products that do not contain nitrosating agents; see DEA.

CA   Oleamidopropyl dimethylamine – synthetic; skin irritant; may be toxic.

†CA   Oleic acid – synthetic; eye, skin, respiratory irritant; may cause acne; low toxicity; CIR says safe as used.

†C   Oleth-n – synthetic; may contain carcinogenic contaminants; limited safety data available; safety determination based upon similar chemicals; not

116

adequately tested; CIR says safe as used for -2, -3, -5, -8, -9, -10, -15, -16, -20, -25, -30; see ethoxylated alcohols.

†C   Oleyl alcohol –synthetic; eye, skin, respiratory irritant; not adequately tested; CIR says safe as used.

SA   Olive oil – may cause acne.

X   o-benzene dicarboxylic acid – synthetic; see phthalic acid.

X   o-nitro-p-aminophenol – synthetic; carcinogen.

X   o-phenylenediamine synthetic; recognized carcinogen by Environmentsl Defense; mutagen.

X   o-phthalic acid – synthetic; see phthalic acid.

*C   Orange bitter – essential oil; phototoxic, do not use for 24 hours prior to going out in sun; see essential oils.

*S   Orange blossom oil – essential oil; see neroli oil.

*S   Orange essence – see orange oil.

*S   Orange oil – essential oil; astringent; antibacterial; skin irritant; may cause photosensitivity; see essential oils.

*C   Oregano oil – essential oil; antiseptic; anti-bacterial; anti-fungal; severe skin irritant; avoid if pregnant or lactating; see essential oils.

*C   Origanum oil – essential oil; see oregano oil.

*C   Origanum compactum – see oregano oil.

*C1   Origanum majorana – essential oil; see marjoram oil.

C   Orris oil – essential oil; purgative; causes asthma, hay fever, stuffy nose, red eyes, infantile eczema, nausea and vomiting; toxic.

CA   Oryzanol – plant derived; may cause contact dermatitis, allergic skin rashes; from rice bran, barley or corn oil; easily absorbed; non-toxic.

C   Other ingredients – ingredients not required to be listed on the label; may or may not be harmful; may be contaminated with carcinogens or other harmful chemicals.

X   Oxirane – synthetic; see ethylene oxide.

CA   Oxybenzone – synthetic; may cause photosensitivity; skin irritant.

117

XA   <u>Oxymethylene</u> – synthetic; see formaldehyde.

CA   <u>PABA</u> – synthetic; component of vitamin B; sunscreen; prevents sunburn and may prevent skin cancer; may cause contact dermatitis and photo sensitivity in sensitive individuals; IARC Group 3.

X   <u>p-acetylphenetidin</u> – synthetic; see phenacetin.

X   <u>Padimate-O</u> – synthetic; see octyl dimethyl PABA.

S   <u>Palm fatty acid</u> – synthetic; irritant; low toxicity; not considered hazardous.

†S   <u>Palm oil</u> – plant derived; no known toxicity; CIR says safe as used.

†S   <u>Palm kernel oil</u> – plant derived; no known toxicity; CIR says safe as used.

*†CA   <u>Palm stearic acid</u> – synthetic; stearic acid derived from palm; see stearic acid.

*C1   <u>Palmarosa oil</u> – essential oil; antiseptic, anti-bacterial; antifungal; antiviral; caution if pregnant; see essential oils.

†C   <u>Palmitate</u> – synthetic; possible skin irritant; adverse reactions.

†CA   <u>Palmitic acid</u> – synthetic; skin, eye, respiratory irritant.

CA   <u>Palmityl alcohol</u> – synthetic; may cause skin, eye, respiratory irritation; see cetyl alcohol.

CA   <u>P-aminobenzoic acid</u> – synthetic; see PABA.

CA   <u>Para aminobenzoic acid</u> – synthetic; see PABA.

C1   <u>Panax ginseng</u> – herb; demulcent; stimulant; may increase cell life; may cause vaginal bleeding; avoid if asthma, cardiac arrhythmia, clotting problems, emphysema, fever, high blood pressure, pregnant; do not give to children.

†S   <u>Panthenol</u> – natural; B vitamin; CIR says safe as used.

†S   <u>Pantothenic acid</u> – natural or synthetic; vitamin B5; beneficial for hair; see nutrient additives CIR says safe as used.

†CA   <u>Parabens</u> – synthetic; derived from petroleum; absorbed through the skin; may irritate skin; may be toxic if swallowed; potential mutagen; endocrine

disrupter; may impair fertility; in recent studies, parabens have been found in breast cancer tumors, but it is unknown if they had a part in causing the tumors; not adequately tested; not recommended for children; CIR is re-evaluating safety, previously considered safe as used.

†C   <u>Paraffin</u> – synthetic; petroleum derivative; may contain carcinogenic contaminants; CIR says safe as used.

†X   <u>Paraphenylenediamine</u> – synthetic; CIR says safe as used; see p-phenylenediamine.

X   <u>Paraphenylenediamine dihydrochloride</u>– synthetic; see phenylenediamine.

CA   <u>Parsley oil</u> – essential oil; skin irritant; toxic in strong doses; stimulates the nervous system; phototoxic; may cause miscarriage.

CA   <u>Parsley seed oil</u> – see parsley oil

*S   <u>Patchouli oil</u> – essential oil; antiseptic; anti-fungal; may irritate the chemically sensitive; see essential oils.

†SA   <u>Peanut oil</u> – plant derived; may cause acne; avoid if peanut allergy; CIR says safe as used.

C   <u>PEG</u> – synthetic polymers of ethylene oxide; eye and skin irritant; hazardous on large areas of the body; many PEG polymers should not be used on damaged skin; may be contaminated with dangerous levels of 1,4-dioxane, a carcinogen; see ethoxylated alcohols; many of the PEG polymers, from PEG-7 to PEG-800, are on the CIR high priority review list.

C   <u>PEG-n (4-200)</u> – synthetic; see PEG.

†C   <u>PEG-4</u> – synthetic; CIR says safe as used; see PEG.

†C   <u>PEG-6</u> – synthetic; CIR panel says safe, but should not be used on damaged skin; see PEG.

†C   <u>PEG-20</u> – synthetic; see PEG-6.

†C   <u>PEG-75</u> – synthetic; see PEG-6.

C   <u>PEG-2M</u> – synthetic; may be contaminated with dangerous levels of 1,4-dioxane, a carcinogen; see ethoxylated alcohols.

C   PEG 90M – synthetic; may be contaminated with dangerous levels of 1,4-dioxane, a carcinogen; see ethoxylated alcohols.

C   PEG-n cocamine – synthetic; CIR panel says insufficient data to support safety.

†CA   PEG-3 Dimethicone – synthetic; see dimethicone copolyol; PEG.

†CA   PEG-7 Dimethicone – synthetic; see dimethicone copolyol; PEG.

†CA   PEG-7 glycerol cocoate – synthetic; see PEG; CIR says safe in rinse-off products and up to 10% in leave-on products.

†CA   PEG-8 Dimethicone – synthetic; see dimethicone copolyol; PEG.

†CA   PEG-9 Dimethicone – synthetic; see dimethicone copolyol; PEG.

†CA   PEG-10 Dimethicone – synthetic; see dimethicone copolyol; PEG.

†CA   PEG-12 Dimethicone – synthetic; see dimethicone copolyol; PEG.

†CA   PEG-14 Dimethicone – synthetic; see dimethicone copolyol; PEG.

†CA   PEG-17 Dimethicone – synthetic; see dimethicone copolyol; PEG.

†CA   PEG-n lanolin – synthetic; CIR says safe as used for -5, -20, -24, -25, -27, -30, -40, -50, -60, -75, -85, -100; see PEG, lanolin.

†C   PEG-n soy sterol – synthetic; CIR panel says safe as used for -5, -10, -16, -25; see PEG, soy.

†C   PEG-n stearate – synthetic; CIR says safe as used for -2, -6, -8, -20, -32, -40, -50, -100, -150;see PEG.

C   PEG/PPG 17/6 copolymer – synthetic; may be contaminated with dangerous levels of 1,4-dioxane, a carcinogen; see ethoxylated alcohols.

†CA   PEG/PPG-3/10 Dimethicone – synthetic; see dimethicone copolyol; PEG.

†CA   PEG/PPG-4/12 Dimethicone – synthetic; see dimethicone copolyol; PEG.

†CA   PEG/PPG-6/11 Dimethicone – synthetic; see dimethicone copolyol; PEG.

†CA   PEG/PPG-8/14 Dimethicone – synthetic; see dimethicone copolyol; PEG.

†CA   PEG/PPG-14/4 Dimethicone – synthetic; see dimethicone copolyol; PEG.

†CA   PEG/PPG-15/15 Dimethicone – synthetic; see dimethicone copolyol; PEG.

†CA   PEG/PPG-16/2 Dimethicone – synthetic; see dimethicone copolyol; PEG.

†CA   PEG/PPG-17/18 Dimethicone – synthetic; see dimethicone copolyol; PEG.

†CA   PEG/PPG-18/18 Dimethicone – synthetic; see dimethicone copolyol; PEG.

†CA   PEG/PPG-19/19 Dimethicone – synthetic; see dimethicone copolyol; PEG.

†CA   PEG/PPG-20/6 Dimethicone – synthetic; see dimethicone copolyol; PEG.

†CA   PEG/PPG-20/15 Dimethicone – synthetic; see dimethicone copolyol; PEG.

†CA   PEG/PPG-20/20 Dimethicone – synthetic; see dimethicone copolyol; PEG.

†CA   PEG/PPG-20/23 Dimethicone – synthetic; see dimethicone copolyol; PEG.

†CA   PEG/PPG-20/29 Dimethicone – synthetic; see dimethicone copolyol; PEG.

†CA   PEG/PPG-22/23 Dimethicone – synthetic; see dimethicone copolyol; PEG.

†CA   PEG/PPG-22/24 Dimethicone – synthetic; see dimethicone copolyol; PEG.

†CA   PEG/PPG-23/6 Dimethicone – synthetic; see dimethicone copolyol; PEG.

†CA   PEG/PPG-25/25 Dimethicone – synthetic; see dimethicone copolyol; PEG.

†CA   PEG/PPG-27/27 Dimethicone – synthetic; see dimethicone copolyol; PEG.

*S   Pelargonium graveolens – essential oil; see geranium oil.

C Pentasodium pentate – synthetic; skin and mucous membrane irritant; on CIR high priority review list.

CA Pentylene glycol – synthetic; derived from petroleum; may cause contact dermatitis; FDA says glycols may cause adverse reactions; low toxicity.

*†C1 Peppermint oil – essential oil; antiseptic; anti-inflammatory; may cause hay fever, skin irritation; frequent use may cause contact sensitization; use with caution or avoid if pregnant or high blood pressure; CIR says safe as used if pulegone constituent is ≤1%; see essential oils.

X Perchloroethylene – synthetic; see tetrachloroethylene.

CA Perfumes – synthetic; may cause skin irritation, headaches, dizziness, coughing, vomiting, hyperpigmentation.

C Persulphates – synthetic; may irritate skin and mucous membranes; may cause sensitization by inhalation or skin contact; contains ammonium salts, see ammonia.

CA Peruvian balsam – plant derived; see balsam of Peru.

X Perylene – contaminant in waxes, mineral oil; not adequately tested; extremely hazardous to the ecosystem; IARC Group 3.

X p-ethoxyacetanilide – synthetic; see phenacetin.

*S Petitgrain – essential oil; antiseptic; anti-bacterial; anti-inflammatory; may cause photosensitivity; see essential oils.

CA Petrolatum – synthetic; petroleum derivative; may contain carcinogenic contaminants; may cause acne; prevents skin from breathing and eliminating waste;may discolor skin; banned from cosmetics in Europe unless manufacturer proves safety.

†CA Petroleum distillates – synthetic; petroleum or coal tar derivative; may mimic estrogen and disturb hormonal balance; CIR says safe as used; see naphtha.

C PG-Hydroxyethylcellulose Cocodimonium Chloride – synthetic; derived from propylene glycol; not adequately tested; not evaluated by CIR

X Phenacetin – synthetic; severe skin irritant; carcinogen, IARC Group 2A; mutagen; toxic if ingested.

X Phenol – synthetic solvent; coal tar derivative; toxic if inhaled, swallowed or absorbed through the skin; ingestion of 1.5 grams or .05 ounce has caused death; absorption through skin can cause death; IARC Group 3.

†CA Phenoxyethanol – synthetic solvent; rose fragrance; eye and skin irritant; non-irritating at 2.2% dilution or less; can cause contact dermatitis; harmful if absorbed through skin, inhaled, swallowed; CIR says safe as used.

†CA 2-phenoxyethanol – synthetic; see phenoxyethanol.

†C Phenyl methyl pyrazolone – synthetic; used in hair dyes; coal tar derivative; irritant; may cause pain, redness and swelling; inhalation may cause headache, shortness of breath, cough, rhinorrhea, bronchospasm, chest pain; adverse reproductive effects in lab animals; CIR says safe as used; not evaluated by IARC.

†C Phenyl trimethicone – synthetic; silicone oil; CIR panel says safe as used in cosmetics; safety determined based on toxicity data for a related chemical; not adequately tested.

XA Phenylenediamine – synthetic; skin irritant; has caused cancer in some lab animals; mutagen; may cause asthma, genetic damage, death; photosensitizer; can be absorbed through the skin.

XA 1,2-phenylenediamine – synthetic; see phenylenediamine.

†XA m-phenylenediamine – synthetic; IARC Group 3; CIR says safe if ≤10% in hair dyes; see phenylenediamine.

XA o-phenylenediamine – synthetic; see phenylenediamine.

†XA   p-phenylenediamine – synthetic; sensitizer; IARC Group 3; CIR says safe as used, but use with henna for temporary tattoos is not approved by FDA; see phenylenediamine.

CA   Phenylformic acid – synthetic; skin irritant, harmful if ingested; see benzoic acid.

XA   Phenylmercuric acetate – synthetic; skin irritant; extremely toxic; contains mercury.

C   Phenylmethanol – synthetic; derived from petroleum; toxic; may cause contact dermatitis; see benzyl alcohol.

*CA   3-Phenylpropenal – synthetic; see cinnamic aldehyde.

*C   Phosphoric acid – synthetic; skin, eye, nose, throat and respiratory irritant; corrosive; skin contact and swallowing are moderately toxic.

X   Phthalates – synthetic; used in nail polish and perfumes; penetration enhancer; EPA classifies as probable carcinogen; mutagenic; may damage kidneys, liver, lungs, male reproductive system in lab animals; suspected endocrine disrupters; may be associated with early puberty in girls; not adequately tested; not required to be listed on the label; banned in Europe; see xenoestrogens.

X   Phthalic acid – synthetic; mucous membrane and skin irritant; see phthalates.

*S   Picea alba – essential oil; see spruce oil.

*S   Picea mariana – essential oil; see spruce oil.

CA   Pigments – insoluble uncertified color additives; most are azo dyes or coal tar dyes which are carcinogenic; e.g. Pigment Red 4.

C1   Pinene – essential oil; skin irritant; constituent of pine oil; see pine oil.

C1   Pine oil – essential oil; antiseptic; anti-bacterial; anti-viral; skin and mucous membrane irritant; can balance blood pressure; helps with mental and emotional fatigue; oils not pure may be adulterated with turpentine; caution if pregnant; see essential oils.

C1   <u>Pinus sylvestris</u> – essential oil; see pine oil.

S   <u>Plantago</u> – herb; astringent, heals allergies and skin.

S   <u>Plantain</u> – herb; astringent, heals allergies and skin.

*S   <u>Pogostemon cablin</u> – essential oil; see patchouli oil.

*S   <u>Pogostemon patchouli</u> – essential oil; see patchouli oil.

C   <u>Polyisobutene</u> – synthetic; petroleum derivative; may cause asphyxiation; "slightly poisonous"; not adequately tested; on CIR high priority review list.

X   <u>Polycyclic aromatic hydrocarbons (PAH)</u> – synthetic; carcinogen.

†CA   <u>Polydimethylsiloxane</u> – synthetic; see dimethicone.

C   <u>Polyether glycol</u> – synthetic; see PEG.

C   <u>Polyethoxylated compounds</u> – synthetic; may contain carcinogen 1,4-dioxane; see ethoxylated alcohols.

†C   <u>Polyethylene</u> – synthetic; petroleum derivative; implants have caused cancer in lab animals; ingestion has caused liver and kidney damage in lab animals; IARC Group 3; not adequately tested; CIR says safe as used.

C   <u>Polyethylene glycol</u> – synthetic; can break down into formaldehyde; see PEG, formaldehyde.

C   <u>Polyglycol</u> – synthetic; see PEG.

CA   <u>Polymethyl methacrylate</u> – synthetic; eye, skin and respiratory irritant; animal studies indicate possible carcinogen; not adequately tested; on CIR high priority list for review; IARC Group 3.

CA   <u>Polyols</u> – synthetic; see polyethylene glycol, propylene glycol.

C   <u>Polyoxethylene compounds</u> – synthetic; may be contaminated with carcinogenic 1,4-dioxane; see ethoxylated alcohols.

C   <u>Polyoxyethylene sorbitan monooleate</u> – synthetic; skin irritant; may be contaminated with carcinogenic 1,4-dioxane; see ethoxylated alcohols.

†CA   <u>Polypropylene glycol</u> – synthetic; petroleum derivative; skin and eye irritant; slightly toxic on skin contact; hazardous on large areas of the body;

CIR panel says safe up to 50% concentration for PPG-9, -12, -15, -17, -20, -26, -30, -34.

†XA Polyquaternium-10 – synthetic; see quaternary ammonium compounds; CIR says safe as used.

†C Polysorbate (1-85) – synthetic; skin irritant; possible sensitizer; not adequately tested; CIR says safe as used for -20, -21, -40, -61, -65, -81, -85.

†C Polysorbate-60 – synthetic; may be contaminated with carcinogen 1,4-dioxane; see ethoxylated alcohols; CIR says safe as used.

†C Polysorbate-80 – synthetic; may be contaminated with carcinogen 1,4-dioxane; see ethoxylated alcohols; CIR says safe as used.

†XA Polyvinyl acetate – synthetic; IARC Group 3; CIR says safe as used; see polyvinylpyrrolidone.

†XA Polyvinylpyrrolidone – synthetic; petroleum derivative; may cause gas, constipation, lung and kidney damage; may cause foreign bodies in lungs from breathing in hairspray containing this ingredient; IARC Group 3; withdrawn from drug use after being found unsafe.

†C Potassium cocohydrolyzed protein – synthetic; animal derivative; contains some processed free glutamic acid (MSG).

X Potassium fluoride – synthetic; toxic; can cause dental fluorosis; corrosive; severe mucous membrane irritant; harmful if absorbed through skin, ingested, inhaled; may cause brain, kidney damage, death; may harm fetus, embryo; IARC Group 3; see fluoride.

X Potassium fluorosilicate – synthetic; toxic; repeated exposure can cause fluoride poisoning; corrosive; severe mucous membrane, eye skin irritant; harmful if absorbed through skin, ingested, inhaled; ingestion may result in convusions, central nervous system depression, kidney damage; not adeaquately tested; IARC Group 3; see fluoride.

C   Potassium hydroxide – synthetic; severe skin and eye irritant; has caused tumors on skin of mice; ingestion can be fatal.

φS   Potassium sodium copper chlorophyllin – plant derived; only for use in toothpaste or tooth powder; must be used according to specific requirements; no short or long term adverse effects were noted in a study on rats.

*†C   Potassium sorbate – synthetic; skin irritant, may be mutagenic; mildly toxic if swallowed; CIR says safe as used.

†C   PPG – synthetic; see polypropylene glycol.

C   PPG-2-isodeceth-4 – synthetic; may contain carcinogenic contaminants; see ethoxylated alcohols.

C   PPG-m ceteth-n – synthetic; may be contaminated with carcinogens; see ethoxylated alcohols.

C   PPG-2 methyl ether – synthetic; skin, eye, respiratory irritant; narcotic in high doses; has caused death in lab animals from skin exposure; on CIR high priority review list; see polypropylene glycol.

C   PPG-2 methyl ether acetate – synthetic; eye and mucous membrane irritant; may cause cough, drowsiness, dizziness; high doses cause central nervous system depression; absorbed through skin; teratogenic in lab animals; not adequately tested; on CIR high priority review list; see polypropylene glycol.

CA   Procaine – synthetic; see novocain.

CA   Procaine hydrochloride – synthetic; see novocain.

*†C   Propane – petroleum derivative; propellant; neurotoxin at high concentrations; flammable; CIR says safe as used.

†CA   1,2-propanediol – synthetic; see polypropylene glycol.

CA   Propanediols – synthetic; skin irritant; causes unilateral pupil dilation; may cause delayed allergic reaction.

*C   1,2,3-propanetriol – see glycerol.

C   Propantheline bromide – synthetic; causes unilateral pupil dilation; adverse effects to reproductive system; not adeqately tested; safety data not available.

†S   Propolis – natural; from bees; skin irritant.

†CA   Propyl gallate – plant derived; skin irritant; may cause contact dermatitis, sensitization; CIR panel says safe if ≤1%; under re-review by CIR.

†CA   Propyl paraben – synthetic; skin irritant; associated with numerous of health problems, including contact dermatitis and asthma; endocrine disrupter; strong allergen; research shows it decreases sperm production; CIR says safe as used, but is re-evaluating safety.

CA   Propyl-p-hydroxybenzoate – synthetic; see propylparaben.

CA   Propylamine – synthetic; causes skin irritation, contact dermatitis.

†CA   Propylene glycol – synthetic; petrochemical, best avoided; absorbs quickly through skin; penetration enhancer; strong irritant; may cause delayed allergic reaction, acne, contact dermatitis; NIOSH says neurotoxin, may cause kidney, liver damage; EPA says not fully investigated for carcinogenic potential; CIR says safe if ≤50%.

C   Propylene glycol ceteth-n – synthetic; may contain carcinogenic contaminants; see ethoxylated alcohols.

C   Propylene glycol-2 myristyl propionate – synthetic; may cause acne; safety data not available.

†CA   Propylparaben – synthetic; preservative; skin irritant; low toxicity; strong allergen; may cause contact dermatitis; see propyl paraben, parabens.

X   Psoralen – plant derived; phototoxic chemical; may damage DNA and cause mutations, tumors or neoplasms.

S   Pure vegetable esters

S   Purified water

†XA   PVP – synthetic; CIR says safe as used; see polyvinylpyrrolidone.

S   Pyridoxine – see vitamin B6.

X   Pyrocatechol – synthetic; CIR panel determined this ingredient to be unsafe for leave-on products; insufficient data available to assure safety for use in hair dyes; IARC Grup 2B.

φC   Pyrophyllite – mineral; aluminum compound of anhydrous aluminum silicate and silica; aluminum has been linked to Alzheimer's; see external use only.

CA   Quaternary ammonium compounds – synthetic; derived from ammonium chloride; caustic; skin and eye irritant; sensitizers; may be toxic; degree of toxicity varies among the different compounds, depends on concentration; cause hair to become dry and brittle with long-term use; may cause anaphalytic shock.

†XA   Quaternarium-15 – synthetic; skin and eye irritant; primary cause of dermatitis related to preservatives in skin care products; sensitizer; releases formaldehyde; may cause birth defects; teratogenic effects in rats; for those extremely sensitive, may cause asthma, respiratory arrest; CIR says safe as used; see formaldehyde.

†CA   Quaternarium-18 – synthetic; skin and eye irritant; sensitizer; see quaternary ammonium compounds; CIR says safe as used.

C   Quinaldine – synthetic; strong mucous membrane irritant; harmful if absorbed through skin; moderate health hazard.

XA   Quinol – synthetic; see hydroquinone.

XA   Quinoline yellow – synthetic; coal tar derivative; skin irritant; causes dermatitis; a carcinogen.

XA   Quinolines – synthetic; derived from coal tar, a carcinogen; skin irritant; causes dermatitis;.

XA   Quinophthalone – synthetic; derived from coal tar; see solvent yellow 33.

C1   Ravensara – essential oil; antiseptic; anti-bacterial; anti-viral; anti-fungal; avoid if pregnant; see essential oils.

C1 <u>Ravensara aromatica</u> – essential oil; see ravensara.

XA <u>Red No. 3</u> – synthetic; coal tar derivative; carcinogen; banned for cosmetics and drugs used externally; still approved for use in foods and drugs taken internally

φXA <u>Red No. 4</u> – synthetic; coal tar derivative; causes atrophied adrenal glands and bladder polyps in animals, banned in food and drugs, but allowed in cosmetics; see external use only

CA <u>Red No. 36</u> – synthetic; azo dye, derived from phenol; skin irritant; causes acne.

φCA <u>Red No. 40</u> – see FD&C Red No. 40.

φCA <u>Red No. 40 Lake</u> – see FD&C Red No. 40 aluminum lake.

†CA <u>Red oil</u> – synthetic; see oleic acid.

CA <u>Red petrolatum</u> – synthetic; petroleum derivative; may cause skin discoloration, photosensitivity; derived from petroleum.

†XA <u>Resorcinol</u> – synthetic; causes contact dermatitis; eye and skin irritant; when using, avoid acne preparations, alcohol-containing products, medicated cosmetics, abrasive cleansers and soaps; endocrine disrupter; FDA states resorcinol not shown safe and effective as claimed in over-the-counter products; IARC Group 3; CIR says safe as used.

X <u>Resorcinolphthalein</u> – synthetic; see fluoresceins.

†*S <u>Retinol</u> – natural; beneficial for skin; see vitamin A; CIR says safe as used.

†S <u>Retinyl palmitate</u> – synthetic; may cause contact dermatitis; see vitamin A; CIR says safe as used.

C <u>Rhodamine B</u> – synthetic; interferes with collagen synthesis on the lips; inhibits cellular metabolism of the skin; has caused cancer in lab animals; no human data available; IARC Group 3.

C <u>Rhodamines</u> – synthetic; inhibits cellular metabolism of the skin.

S <u>Riboflavin</u> – natural; see vitamin B2.

*CA   Ricinoleamidopropyl dimethylamine lactate – synthetic; corrosive to skin, eyes, throat, nose; toxic by skin contact and if swallowed.

SA   Ricinoleic acid – synthetic; skin irritant; purgative; may cause dermatitis;component of castor oil.

SA   Ricinus oil – plant derived; see castor oil.

*C1   Rosa damascena – essential oil; see rose oil.

S   Rosa rubiginosa – carrier oil; see rosehip oil.

S   Rosalina – essential oil; anti-bacterial; anti-fungal; heating causes loss of therapeutic value; considered safe, but not formally tested; see essential oils.

*C1   Rose oil – essential oil; anti-infectious; aphrodisiac; use cautiously or avoid if pregnant; see essential oils.

*C1   Rose centifolia – essential oil; see rose oil.

*C1   Rose damascena – essential oil; see rose oil.

C1   Rose geranium oil – essential oil; potential mild skin irritant; avoid if epileptic, pregnant.

S   Rosehip oil – carrier oil; healing for skin conditions; may aggravate acne.

*C1   Rosemarinus officinalis – essential oil; see rosemary oil.

*C1A   Rosemary extract – plant derived; may cause skin irritation, photosensitivity; avoid if pregnant, epileptic, high blood pressure; see extract.

*C1   Rosemary oil – essential oil; antiseptic; astringent; avoid if pregnant, epileptic, high blood pressure; see essential oils.

*S   Rosewood – see rosewood oil

*S   Rosewood oil – essential oil; anti-bacterial; anti-viral; anti-fungal; non-toxic; non-sensitizing; may irritate sensitive skin; see essential oils.

CA   Rosin – natural extract; skin irritant; may cause dermatitis.

*C1   Rosmarinus officinalis – essential oil; see rosemary oil.

C   Rue oil – essential oil; eye, skin, mucous membrane irritant; large amounts have caused poisoning; may cause photosensitivity; should not be used by pregnant, nursing women and those under 18 years.

X   Saccharin – synthetic; potential carcinogen; has caused cancer in lab animals; NTP has delisted saccharin as a carcinogen and removed warning labels; IARC has down graded it to Group 3; however, there are still scientists and groups like Center for Science in the Public Interest who believe that saccharin should be listed as a carcinogen due to its ability to cause cancer in animals.

*†C   Safflower oil – plant derived; deep moisturizer; may irritate skin; may cause acne; see oils: CIR says safe as used.

C   Sage – herb; astringent; antiseptic; disinfectant; avoid if pregnant, epileptic, high blood pressure.

*C1   Sage oil – essential oil; astringent; antiseptic; disinfectant; avoid if pregnant, epileptic, high blood pressure; toxic if taken internally; see essential oils.

C1A   St. Johnswort – herb; see hypericum perforatum.

†C   Salicylic acid – synthetic; eye and skin irritant; poison if swallowed; large amounts absorbed through skin may cause abdominal pain, vomiting, tinnitis, mental disturbances; mutagen; CIR says safe as used.

*C1   Salvia officinalis – essential oil; see sage oil.

*C1   Salvia sclarea – essential oil; see clary sage.

*S   Sandalwood oil – essential oil; antiseptic; astringent; see essential oils.

*S   Santalum album – essential oil; see sandalwood oil.

C   Sassafras oil - essential oil; toxic; suspected carcinogen.

*C   Satureja montana – essential oil; see mountain savory.

CA   Scoparone – synthetic; see coumarin.

CA   Scotch pine – herb; essential oil; fragrance; skin irritant; may cause sensitization.

C   SD alcohol – synthetic solvent; see denatured alcohol.

C   SD alcohol 40 – synthetic solvent; see denatured alcohol.

C   SD alcohol 40 – 8 – synthetic solvent; see denatured alcohol.

S   Seed of plantago – herb, antibacterial, anti-fungal.

C   Selenium – trace mineral essential to health in very small doses; excess amounts cause selenium toxicity; acute exposure may cause diarrhea, nausea, vomiting; chronic exposure may affect the nervous system; not adequately tested for effects from skin absorption; IARC Group 3.

C   Selenium sulfide – synthetic; severe eye and skin irritant; EPA says probable carcinogen; IARC Group 3.

†S   Sesame oil – plant derived; may cause acne; see oils; CIR says safe as used.

CA   Sesquiterpine lactone – synthetic; naturally occurring component of essential oils; may cause severe allergies.

†CA   Shellac – animal derived; resin secreted by insects; used in mascara; may cause contact dermatitis; not adequately tested; CIR says safe if ≤6%.

C   Silica – mineral; toxic if inhaled; skin and eye irritant; may be contaminated with crystalline quartz, a carcinogen; synthetic amorphous fumed silica may be free of crystalline quartz; absorbs moisture; drying to the skin; see external use only; on CIR high priority list for review.

S   Silicates – most abundant class of minerals, composed of silicon, oxygen and a metal; no known toxicity.

CA   Silicones – synthetic polymers; not absorbed through the skin; may irritate skin, eyes; may cause sensitization; some silicones may cause adverse effects, including harm to the kidneys and liver; have caused toxicity and immune dysfunction in many women with breast implants; for external use only.

CA   Silk powder – natural; may cause hives; systemic symptoms if ingested or inhaled.

φC   Silver – metal; mucous membrane and skin irritant; skin discoloration may result from prolonged absorption; limited to fingernail polish.

XA   Soapstone – natural strone comprised mostly of talc; see talc.

†CA   Sodium benzoate – synthetic; skin irritant; toxic if swallowed; avoid if asthma or liver problems; may cause hyperactivity in children; associated with numerous health issues; CIR panel says safe in concentrations up to 5%, insufficient data to support safety in products where exposure involves inhalation.

†*XA   Sodium bisulfite – synthetic; strong skin, eye and mucous membrane irritant; corrosive; mutagen; may cause asthma, anaphylactic shock; contains ammonium salts, see ammonia.

†CA   Sodium carboxymethyl cellulose – synthetic; see cellulose gum.

*S   Sodium chloride – natural; eye and skin irritant.

*CA   Sodium citrate – synthetic; see citric acid.

†C   Sodium cocoyl isethionate – synthetic; eye and skin irritant; slightly to practically nontoxic; CIR says safe at ≤50% in rinse-off products and ≤17% in leave-on products.

†C   Sodium cocoyl sarcosinate – synthetic surfactant; CIR panel says safe in "rinse-off" products as used, safe in "leave-on" products up to 5% concentration, insufficient data to determine safety in products where ingredient may be inhaled, may cause formation of carcinogenic nitrosamines in products containing nitrogen compounds.

*C   Sodium dioctyl sulfosuccinate – synthetic; skin, eye and respiratory irritant; harmful if absorbed through skin, inhaled; harmful if ingested; moderately toxic.

CA   Sodium dodecyl sulfate – synthetic; skin irritant; may cause eczema; contains ammonium salts, see ammonia.

†CA   Sodium dodecylbenzene sulfonate – synthetic; skin and eye irritant; has caused liver, kidney and

134

intestinal damage when ingested by animals; CIR says safe as used.

X   <u>Sodium fluoride</u> – synthetic; poison; severe skin, eye, respiratory irritant; inhalation, ingestion may cause death; toxic effects may be delayed; IARC Group 3; see fluoride.

X   <u>Sodium fluorosilicate</u> – synthetic; health hazard; severe skin, eye, respiratory irritant; may cause nervous, cardiac disorders, bone fluorosis; ingestion may cause convulsions, coma, death; IARC Group 3; see fluoride.

CA   <u>Sodium hyaluronate</u> – found in human cells; may be derived from plant or bird sources or produced synthetically; non-toxic; on CIR high priority review list.

X   <u>Sodium hydroxide</u> – synthetic; severe eye and skin irritant; corrosive; mutagen.

XA   <u>Sodium hydroxymethylglycinate</u> – synthetic; skin and eye irritant; sensitizer; derived from glycine; formaldehyde releaser; breaks down in aqueous solution to sodium glycinate and formaldehyde; formaldehyde is IARC Group 1.

|C   <u>Sodium laureth sulfate</u> – synthetic surfactant; skin and eye irritant; may cause dermatitis; may be contaminated with dangerous levels of toxins; penetration enhancer; see ethoxylated alcohols, CIR says safe as used.

†C   <u>Sodium laureth-n sulfate</u> – synthetic; see sodium laureth sulfate.

C   <u>Sodium Lauroamphoacetate</u> – synthetic; not assessed by CIR; safety data not available; not adequately tested

†C   <u>Sodium lauroyl sarcosinate</u> – synthetic; penetration enhancer; may cause formation of carcinogenic nitrosamines on skin or in body if nitrosating agents present; CIR says safe as used in rinse-off products, but ≤5% with leave-on products; insufficient data to determine safety for products likely to be inhaled.

†CA Sodium lauryl sulfate – synthetic surfactant; may cause dry skin, eczema; eye and skin irritant; inhibits DNA synthesis; potential mutagen; CIR panel says safe for use in "rinse-off" products, up to 1% concentration in "leave-on" products.

X Sodium monofluorophosphate – synthetic; toxic; IARC Group 3; see fluoride.

†C Sodium myreth sulfate – synthetic surfactant; eye and skin irritant; similar to sodium laureth sulfate; CIR says safe as used.

C Sodium oleth sulfate – synthetic; may be contaminated with dangerous levels of toxins; contains ammonium salts; see ammonia, ethoxylated alcohols.

†C Sodium PCA – synthetic; see NaPCA.

C Sodium phosphate – synthetic; skin and eye irritant; may cause dermatitis.

X Sodium saccharin – synthetic; see saccharin.

C Sodium silicate – synthetic; skin, eye and mucous membrane irritant; corrosive; poison if swallowed.

†CA Sodium stearate – synthetic surfactant; 93% stearic acid; see stearic acid; CIR says safe as used.

†C Sodium sulfate – synthetic; skin eye and respiratory irritant; corrosive; may trigger asthma attacks; CIR says safe for rinse-off products and a maximum concentration of 1% in leave-on products; contains ammonium salts, see ammonia.

C Sodium trideceth sulfate – synthetic; may be contaminated with dangerous levels of toxins; see ethoxylated alcohols; contains ammonium salts, see ammonia.

*X Sodiumsulphosuccinate – synthetic; eye, mucous membrane and skin irritant; potentially harmful if absorbed through skin, inhaled or swallowed; not adequately tested.

CA Solvent dyes – synthetic; uncertified colors; most are azo dyes or coal tar dyes which are carcinogenic; e.g. Solvent Green 3.

XA   Solvent yellow 33 – synthetic; coal tar dye; sensitizer; see D&C Yellow No. 11, quinolines.

†C   Sorbic acid – synthetic; causes hives; skin irritant; mutagen; has caused cancer in lab animals; mildly toxic if swallowed; CIR says safe as used.

†C   Sorbitan isostearate – synthetic; skin irritant; CIR says safe as used.

†C   Sorbitan laurate – synthetic; may cause hives; carcinogenic in one aminal study; CIR says safe as used.

†C   Sorbitan oleate – synthetic; causes hives; lab studies show it interferes with DNA repair after UV exposure; CIR says safe as used; safety determined based upon toxicity data for a related chemical.

†S   Sorbitan olivate – synthetic; derived from olive oil; CIR says safe as used.

†C   Sorbitan palmitate – synthetic; may cause hives; CIR says safe as used; safety determined based upon toxicity data for a related chemical.

†CA   Sorbitan sesquioleate – synthetic; may cause hives; CIR says safe as used; safety determined based upon toxicity data for a related chemical.

†C   Sorbitan stearate – synthetic; may cause hives; CIR says safe as used; safety determined based upon toxicity data for a related chemical.

*CA   Sorbitol – natural; may be natural or chemically derived; no known toxicity for external use; taken internally, may cause gastrointestinal distress, may change rate of absorption of drugs; safety data not available for long-term exposure.

CA   Soy oil – plant derived; absorbed through the skin; may be genetically modified; may cause allergic acne.

CA   Soy protein – synthetic; may be genetically modified; may cause allergic acne; may contain MSG or processed free glutamic acid.

CA   Soyamide DEA – synthetic; soy may be genetically modified; see DEA.

CA   Soybean oil – plant derived; see soy oil.

*C1   <u>Spearmint oil</u> – essential oil; antiseptic; anti-bacterial; anti-fungal; avoid on infants and small children; use cautiously or avoid if pregnant; see essential oils.

*C1   <u>Spikenard</u> – essential oil; skin tonic; anti-bacterial, anti-fungal; avoid if pregnant.

*S   <u>Spruce oil</u> – essential oil; anti-inflammatory; anti-infectious; disinfectant; see essential oils.

†CA   <u>Squalane</u> – plant, animal or synthetically derived; hydrogenated; penetrates skin deeply; may irritate eye, skin, respiratory tract; not adequately tested; CIR says safe as used.

†C   <u>Squalene</u> – plant or animal derived; naturally present in human sebum; potential skin, eye, respiratory irritant; may be harmful if absorbed through skin, inhaled or ingested; toxicological properties unknown; CIR says safe as used.

X   <u>Stannous fluoride</u> – synthetic; corrosive; toxic on skin contact, if ingested or inhaled; IARC Group 3; see fluoride.

CA   <u>Starch</u> – plant derived; may cause stuffy nose if inhaled; blocks pores on skin.

†C   <u>Stearalkonium hectorite</u> – synthetic; may be contaminated with carcinogenic contaminants; may form nitrosamines on skin or after absorbed; CIR says safe as used.

CA   <u>Stearamidoethyl diethylamine phosphate</u> – synthetic; skin and mucous membrane irritant.

CA   <u>Stearamidopropyl dimethylamine</u> – synthetic; skin and mucous membrane irritant; may be carcinogenic.

C   <u>Stearamin oxyd</u> – synthetic; may cause formation of carcinogenic nitrosamines.

†C   <u>Stearamine oxide</u> – synthetic; may cause formation of carcinogenic nitrosamines; CIR panel says safe for "rinse-off" products and up to 5% concentration in "leave-on" products.

†C   <u>Steareth-n</u> – synthetic; may be contaminated with dangerous levels of toxins; see ethoxylated alcohols; CIR says safe as used for -2, -10, -15, -20.

138

*†CA   Stearic acid – synthetic; skin irritant; potential sensitizer; may cause acne; CIR says safe as used; safety determined based upon toxicity data for a related chemical.

†CA   Stearyl alcohol – synthetic; skin irritant; may cause contact dermatitis; CIR says safe as used; safety determined based upon toxicity data for a related chemical.

XA   Steatite – natural stone; contains up to 50% talc; see talc.

C   Stinging nettle – herb; see nettle.

*S   Styrax benzoin – essential oil; see benzoin.

C   Sucrose cocoate – synthetic surfactant; safety data not available.

†C   Sugar cane extract – natural extract; see alpha hydroxy acids.

CA   Sulfanilamide – antibacterial; toxic; eye, skin, respiratory irritant; harmful if inhaled or ingested; classified as a drug; safety not tested for pregnant, breastfeeding women, children and older adults.

CA   Sulfur – mineral; skin, eye and respiratory irritant; banned in products for cold sores, fever blisters and diaper rash; FDA says not shown safe in products for treating lice, poison oak, poison ivy and poison sumac.

†C   Sulisobenzone – synthetic; see benzophenone.

S   Sunflower oil – plant derived; see oils.

C1   Sweet birch oil – essential oil; see birch oil.

*C1   Sweet fennel oil – essential oil; anti-inflammatory; antiseptic; diuretic; skin sensitizer; epileptics should not use; avoid during pregnancy.

*S   Sweet orange oil – essential oil; see orange oil.

C   Symphytum officinalis – herb; see comfrey.

φC   Synthetic iron oxides – slight eye and skin irritant; see iron oxides.

XA   Talc – natural mineral; possible skin and lung irritant; toxic if inhaled; carcinogen, IARC Group 1 if contains asbestiform fibers, IARC Group 3 if it does not contain asbestiform fibers; quantity of asbestiform fibers in cosmetic-grade talc is unregulated in U.S.; never use on babies; on CIR high priority list for review.

XA Talcum – see talc.

XA Talcum powder – synthetic; may cause vomiting, coughing, pneumonia in babies if inhaled; increases risk of ovarian cancer if used on sanitary napkins or genitals; see talc.

C1 Tanacetum vulgare – essential oil; see wild tansy oil.

*S Tangerine oil – essential oil; anti-inflammatory; may cause photosensitivity; irritate eyes and skin.

*C1 Tarragon oil – essential oil; antiseptic; anti-bacterial; anti-viral; avoid if pregnant, epileptic; see essential oils.

†C TEA – synthetic; skin, mucous membrane and eye irritant; causes contact dermatitis; sensitizer; may cause formation of carcinogenic nitrosamines in products containing nitrogen compounds; may contain nitrosamine contaminants not listed on the label; mildly toxic if swallowed; not adequately tested; CIR says safe in rinse-off products, up to 5% concentration in leave-on products, and should not be used in products containing N-nitrosating agents; IARC Group 3.

C TEA carbomer – synthetic; see TEA.

†C TEA coco hydrolyzed protein – synthetic; severe skin irritant; contains processed free glutamic acid (MSG); CIR says safe as used; see TEA, MSG.

C TEA cocoyl glutamate – synthetic; see TEA, glutamic acid.

†C TEA lauryl sulfate – synthetic surfactant; contains ammonium salts; see ammonia, TEA, sodium lauryl sulfate; CIR says safe if ≤10.5%.

C TEA salicylate – synthetic; phototoxic chemical; in sunlight may cause formation of carcinogenic nitrosamines; see salicylic acid, TEA.

†CA TEA stearate – synthetic; see TEA, stearic acid; CIR says safe in reinse-off products, ≤15% in leave-on products, and NOT used with N-nitrosating agents.

*S   Tea tree oil – essential oil; see melaleuca alternifolia.

†CA   Tegobetaine L7 – synthetic; see cocamidopropyl betaine.

†CA   Tektamer 38 – synthetic; see methyldibromo glutaronitrile.

C   Tergitol – synthetic; skin, eye, respiratory irritant; skin contact may cause pain and redness; endocrine disrupter; not adequately tested; safety determined based upon toxicity data for a related chemical.

CA   Terpenes – hydrocarbons, like petroleum products, mineral oil, paraffin, ozokerite; may cause facial psoriasis.

CA   2-tert-butylhydroquinone – synthetic; can cause contact dermatitis.

XA   Tertiary ammonium compounds – synthetic; skin irritant; may cause anaphylactic shock

X   Tetrachloroethylene – synthetic; skin, eye and respiratory irritant; dries skin; neurotoxin; probable carcinogen, IARC Group 2A.

CA   1-tetradecanol – synthetic; see myristyl alcohol.

CA   Tetrahydronaphthalene – synthetic; skin, eye and respiratory irritant; may cause severe dermatitis, liver and kidney damage; central nervous system depressant; neurotoxin.

X   2,4,5,7-tetraiodofluorescein disodium salt – synthetic; coal tar color; carcinogen.

†CA   Tetrasodium EDTA – synthetic; penetration enhancer; see disodium EDTA; taken orally can cause calcium depletion, gastrointestinal discomfort; overexposure may cause skin, eye, respiratory irritation; CIR says safe as used.

CA   Tetrasodium salt – synthetic; see disodium EDTA.

SA   Theobroma oil – plant derived; see cocoa butter.

†XA   Thioglycolic acid – synthetic; harmful; severe allergen, skin irritant; causes hair to break; requires a warning on the label in Europe; CIR says safe if ≤15.4% and avoid or minimize skin exposure; see ammonium thioglycolate.

X   Thiomersal – synthetic; preservative in eye cosmetics and vaccines given to infants; skin irritant; contains mercury, which has been banned in cosmetics except in eye cosmetics because of mercury buildup; small amounts ingested can be fatal.

C1   Thyme extract – plant derived; skin and mucous membrane irritant; may cause hay fever; avoid if pregnant, high blood pressure, thyroid problems.

*C1   Thyme oil – essential oil; antiseptic; antibacterial, anti-viral; anti-fungal; skin and mucous membrane irritant; avoid if pregnant, high blood pressure, thyroid problems; see essential oils.

*C1   Thymus vulgaris – essential oil; see thyme oil.

φC   Titanium dioxide – synthetic; may irritate skin, eyes; inhalation of large amounts of titanium dioxide dust may cause lung damage; IARC Group 3; not clear if coarse or fine particles are absorbed through the skin; may generate free radicals when exposed to sunlight; excess free radicals are associated with cancer; micronized titanium dioxide can penetrate the cells, cause cell damage and should be avoided; not adequately tested; not evaluated by CIR.

†CA   Tocopherol (vitamin E) – natural or synthetic; antioxidant; healing to skin; may cause contact dermatitis; may be soy, peanut, corn based; may be contaminated with hydroquinone; see hydroquinone, nutrient additives; CIR says safe as used.

CA   Tocopherol acetate (vitamin E) – synthetic; may be contaminated with hydroquinone; see hydroquinone, tocopherol.

†CA   Tocopheryl acetate (vitamin E) – synthetic; longer shelf life, but cannot be utilized by the skin; may be contaminated with hydroquinone; see hydroquinone; CIR says safe as used.

†C   Toluene – synthetic; coal tar derivative; skin, eye and respiratory irritant; neurotoxin; may cause asthma and trigger attacks; high concentrations may cause death; repeated inhalation may cause

permanent brain damage; adverse effects worsened if consume alcohol at time of exposure, or suffer from kidney, liver or skin disorders; classified as hazardous by OSHA; IARC Group 3; CIR panel says safe as used in cosmetics.

X   Toluene-2,4-diamine – synthetic; see 2,4-diaminotoluene.

X   2,4-toluenediamine – synthetic; see 2,4-diaminotoluene.

X   m-toluenediamine - synthetic; mutagen, carcinogen.

†CA   Toluenesulfonamide formaldehyde resin – synthetic; skin irritant; strong sensitizer when liquid; causes contact dermatitis.

CA   Tonka bean – plant derived; see coumarin.

CA   Tonka bean camphor – plant derived; see coumarin.

XA   Tricetylmonium chloride – synthetic; see quaternary ammonium compounds.

X   Trichloroethane – synthetic; eye, skin and mucous membrane irritant; neurotoxin; not adequately tested for carcinogenicity; narcotic in high amounts; may adversely affect the heart, including cardiac arrest.

X   1,1,1-tricholorethane – synthetic; see tricholorethane.

CA   Triclosan – synthetic; antibacterial/antimicrobial, not antibiotic, but acts like antibiotic in way it targets bacteria; may kill healthy bacteria as well as harmful bateria; eye, skin and respiratory irritant; may cause contact dermatitis, liver damage; may be contaminated with carcinogenic dioxin; possible endocrine disrupter; moderately toxic on skin contact and if swallowed; high levels have been detected in human breast milk; stored in body fat; classified as a drug by the FDA; no scientific evidence showing it prevents infection; not adequately tested.

†C   Triethanolamine – synthetic; see TEA.

C   Triethanolamine salts – synthetic; eye and skin irritant; see TEA.

†X   <u>Triisopropanolamine</u> – synthetic; severe eye, skin, mucous membrane, upper respiratory tract irritant; harmful if absorbed through skin, inhaled or swallowed; not adequately tested; CIR panel says safe but should not be used in products containing N-nitrosating agents.

X   <u>4,5,8-trimethylpsoralen</u> – synthetic; phototoxic chemical, may damage DNA and cause mutations, tumors or neoplasms; IARC Group 3.

†C   <u>Tri-alpha hydroxy fruit acids</u> – synthetic combined with natural extracts; see alpha hydroxy acids.

†C   <u>Triple fruit acid</u> – synthetic combined with natural extracts;see alpha hydroxy acids.

C   <u>Tropaeolum majus</u> – herb; antibacterial; antifungal; see Indian cress.

XA   <u>Turpentine oil</u> – natural extract; nose, throat and skin irritant; may cause headaches, hallucinations, kidney and lung damage, death; depresses central nervous system.

X   <u>Ultrafine minerals</u> – minerals; see micronized minerals.

X   <u>Ultrafine titanium dioxide</u> – minerals; see micronized titanium dioxide.

φC   <u>Ultramarine blue</u> – natural or synthetic; mineral derived pigment; considered nontoxic; long-term safety data not available; see "external use only."

φC   <u>Ultramarine green</u> – natural or synthetic; mineral derived pigment; considered nontoxic; long-term safety data not available; see "external use only."

φC   <u>Ultramarine pink</u> – natural or synthetic; mineral derived pigment; considered nontoxic; long-term safety data not available; see "external use only."

φC   <u>Ultramarine red</u> – natural or synthetic; mineral derived pigment; considered nontoxic; long-term safety data not available; see "external use only."

φC   <u>Ultramarine violet</u> – natural or synthetic; mineral derived pigment; considered nontoxic; long-term safety data not available; see "external use only."

C   Ultrasomes – bio-engineered enzymes (genetically modified); slow-acting enzymes used in antiaging products for skin repair, moisturizing; deliver cosmetic ingredients to the horny layer of the skin; experimental; safety data not available.

C   Undecylenoyl glycine – synthetic; fatty acid from coconut similar to naturally occurring substances in living organisms; not evaluated by CIR; safety data not available.

*CA   Urea – natural, but usually synthetically produced; skin irritant; mutagen.

X   Urocanic acid – synthetic; phototoxin; not adequately tested; avoid if using alpha-hydroxy acids; CIR panel says insufficient data to support safety.

C   Urtica dioica – essential oil; see nettle.

S   Usnea barbata – botanical; see lichen.

C   Vaccinium myrtillus – herb; see bilberry.

C   Valerates – synthetic; skin irritant; suspected carcinogen.

*C1   Valerian oil – essential oil; anti-bacterial; central nervous system depressant; frequent use may cause contact sensitization, avoid if pregnant; see essential oils.

*C1   Valeriana officinalis – essential oil; see valerian oil.

C   Valeric acid – plant derived; eye, throat, nose and skin irritant; moderately toxic if inhaled or swallowed.

C   Vanillin – synthetic; skin irritant; sensitizer; causes burning sensation, contact dermatitis, eczema, skin pigmentation.

CA   Vegetable emulsifying wax – plant derived; safety data not available.

C   Verbena oil – plant derived; causes photosensitivity; see oils.

*C1   Vetiver oil – essential oil; antiseptic; use cautiously or avoid if pregnant; see essential oils.

*C1   Vetiveria zizanoides – essential oil; see veviter oil.

C   <u>Vinyl acetate/crotonic acid/vinyl neodecanoate polymer</u> – synthetic; toxic if inhaled

C   <u>Violet oil</u> – essential oil; antiseptic; anti-inflammatory; sensitizer; high doses can cause diarrhea and vomiting.

*C   <u>Vitamin A</u> – synthetic; chemically processed; important for the health of the skin; too much can be toxic; see nutrient additives, vitamins.

C   <u>Vitamin B2</u> – synthetic; chemically processed; important for healthy tissues and skin; see nutrient additives, vitamins.

C   <u>Vitamin B3</u> – synthetic; chemically processed; increases circulation; helpful for skin rashes; see nutrient additives, vitamins.

C   <u>Vitamin B6</u> – synthetic; chemically processed; helpful for skin disorders; see nutrient additives, vitamins.

C   <u>Vitamin C</u> – synthetic; chemically processed; antioxidant; preservative; can enhance mineral absorption, can inhibit nitrosamine formation; may be corn based; see nutrient additives, vitamins.

C   <u>Vitamin C palmitate</u> – synthetic; chemically processed; see ascorbic acid, nutrient additives, vitamins.

C   <u>Vitamin D</u> – synthetic; chemically processed; may be helpful to the skin; high doses taken internally can be toxic; see nutrient additives, vitamins.

C   <u>Vitamin E</u> – synthetic; extracted using toxic chemical solvents; antioxidant; heals and protects skin; see nutrient additives, vitamins.

C   <u>Vitamin E acetate</u> – synthetic; extracted using toxic chemical solvents; antioxidant; see vitamin E, nutrient additives, vitamins.

C   <u>Vitamin E linoleate</u> – synthetic; extracted using toxic chemical solvents; antioxidant, moisturizer; see vitamin E, nutrient additives; vitamins.

C   <u>Vitamins</u> – mostly synthetic; "chemically extracted, bio-engineered or isolated, refined/bleached, standardized, stabilized/preserved;" ***derived from*** means processed and synthetic; natural if dehydrated or freeze-dried. Quality and effectiveness may vary depending upon manufacturer; clinically, I've seen great benefit from both high quality USP grade as well as natural; quality is important; avoid bio-engineered/genetically modified.

S   <u>Vitis vinifera extract</u> – plant derived; grape seed extract; therapeutic benefits; antioxidant.

†S   <u>Wheat germ oil</u> – plant derived.

C   <u>Wheat protein</u> – may contain MSG or processed free glutamic acid.

S   <u>Whole grape extract</u> – plant derived; therapeutic benefits.

CA   <u>Wild geranium oil</u> – essential oil; antiseptic; anti-inflammatory; see geranium oil.

S   <u>Wild pansy extract</u> – essential oil; astringent; analgesic; anti-inflammatory; anti-oxidant.

C1   <u>Wild tansy oil</u> – essential oil; anti-bacterial; anti-viral; anti-fungal; not recommended to take internally; avoid if pregnant; see essential oils.

*C1   <u>Wild thyme oil</u> – essential oil; antiseptic; mucous membrane irritant; avoid if pregnant.

†C   <u>Wild yam extract</u> – plant derived; CIR panel says insufficient data to support safety.

C   <u>Wintergreen oil</u> – synthetic; see methyl salicylate.

CA   <u>Witch hazel</u> – herb; anti-inflammatory; astringent; skin irritant; see ethyl alcohol.

X   <u>Wood alcohol</u> – synthetic; see methyl alcohol.

*C   <u>Xanthan gum</u> – natural; may cause eye and skin irritation; potentially harmful if absorbed through skin, inhaled or ingested; extracted with toxic organic solvents; solvent residue may remain in the product; contains "approved" levels of lead and arsenic; not adequately tested.

C   <u>Xanthene</u> – synthetic; interferes with cellular activity; may cause acne.

X   <u>Xylene</u> – hydrocarbon; derived from coal tar, wood tar or petroleum; skin and eye irritant; toxic if inhaled or ingested; neurotoxin; possible teratogen;

carcinogenicity needs to be investigated; not adequately tested; IARC Group 3.

C1   <u>Yarrow extract</u> – herb; CIR panel says insufficient data to support safety; see yarrow oil.

C1   <u>Yarrow oil</u> – essential oil; antiseptic; anti-inflammatory; frequent use may cause contact sensitization; use cautiously or avoid if pregnant; see essential oils.

C   <u>Yeast extract</u> – natural; hidden source of MSG or processed free glutamic acid.

XA   <u>Yellow No. 5 Lake</u> – synthetic; coal tar dye; see FD&C Yellow No. 5 Lake.

XA   <u>Yellow No. 6 Lake</u> – synthetic; coal tar dye; see FD&C Yellow No. 6 Lake.

XA   <u>Yellow No. 11</u> – synthetic; coal tar dye; see D&C yellow No. 11.

C   <u>Ylang ylang oil</u> – essential oil; antiseptic; may cause nausea or headache with long-term use; frequent use may cause contact sensitization; see essential oils.

X   <u>Z-Cote</u> – microfine zinc oxide; particle size <.2 microns; see micronized minerals.

φC   <u>Zinc oxide</u> – synthetic; zinc is an essential mineral, but can have adverse effects if used in excess; may generate free radicals when exposed to sunlight; excess free radicals are associated with cancer; not clear if coarse or fine particles are absorbed through skin; astringent, avoid if dry skin; respiratory irritant; swallowing may cause gastrointestinal upset; do not use on children with skin allergies; avoid micronized zinc oxide; not adequately tested.

†C   <u>Zinc phenolsulfate</u> – synthetic; skin irritant; adversely affected liver, brain and testes in lab animals; contains ammonium salts, see ammonia.

C   <u>Zingiber officinale</u> – essential oil; see ginger oil.

C   <u>Zirconium chlorohydrate</u> – synthetic; skin irritant.

C   <u>Zirconyl chloride</u> – synthetic; skin irritant; moderately toxic if swallowed.

Choosing Safe & Healthy Products

The products listed here were chosen because they are the best I found on the market. I personally, examined every label of every product in this list to make sure that this list included only the safest products on the market.

Originally I planned to include only those products that were 100% natural. But as it is true that not all natural ingredients are safe and healthy, also not all synthetic ingredients are unsafe or harmful. So, the products in this list range from mostly natural to 100% natural and 100% organic.

Since there are no official definitions for natural and synthetic within the cosmetic industry, I have used the definitions for natural and synthetic from the National Organic Program (NOP). They are the standard definitions accepted within the organic foods industry. See page 45.

Even though all the products listed here are, in my opinion, the safest on the market, it's always wise to read labels before you buy because:

- You must decide for yourself if the safety of the ingredients in the products you choose measures up to the standards of safety you want for yourself.
- You might be sensitive to certain ingredients. Even though they might be healthy for most people, they wouldn't be healthy for you and you wouldn't want to use products containing ingredients to which you react.
- Manufacturers sometimes change the ingredients in their products. The ingredients in the product you buy might be different from what was on the label when it was evaluated.
- Reading labels is a good habit to develop, whether it's for cosmetics and personal care products, food, nutritional supplements, medications or household and gardening products. When you're in the habit of reading

labels, you'll be much more likely to avoid buying products with harmful ingredients.

- No matter what the packaging of a product says about the product – it's very often misleading – you can't tell how healthy a product is unless you read and understand the complete list of ingredients.

Not every product of every company listed here is included. So, be sure you read the labels of the products not listed here to make sure they meet your safety requirements.

It's highly likely, that I didn't find all the products on the market that should be included on this list. So, you may find products that you believe are worthy of being included here but are not. By reading the label you can determine for yourself if that's a healthy choice for you. Also you can go to www.dyingtolookgood.com and let me know about healthy products you find, get updates and new information, ask questions and find special discounts on healthy products.

The Products Recommended Here *DO NOT* Contain:

Amino acids
Ammonium laureth sulfate
Ammonium lauryl sulfate
Benzophenones
Benzylhemiformal
BHT or BHA
Carrageenan
Coal tar derivatives
DEA (diethanolamine)
Diazolidinyl urea
DMDM hydantoin
Fluorides
Formaldehyde
Germall 115
Germall II
Homosalate
Hydrolyzed protein

Hydrogenated oils
Imidazolidinyl urea
MEA (monoethanolamine)
4-methyl-benzylidene camphor (4-MBC)
Micronized minerals
Mineral oil
Nayad
Octyl-dimethyl-PABA
Octyl-methoxycinnamate
Padimate-O
Parabens (butyl-, ethyl-, methyl-, propyl-)
PEG
Petrolatum
Propylene glycol
Processed proteins
PVP/VA copolymer
Quaternium-15
Quaternium-18
Silicones
Sodium hydroxymethyl glycinate
Sodium laureth sulfate
Sodium lauryl sulfate
Stearalkonium chloride
Synthetic fragrance
Synthetic colors, FD&C, D&C., Ext. D&C colors
Talc
TEA (triethanolamine)
Yeast extract

Codes After Some Product Names

There are some products in the Healthy Products list that
contain
- grapefruit seed extract
- titanium dioxide
- zinc oxide

Because these ingredients are controversial, (see pages 28 and 38), I have identified the products containing these ingredients for those who want to avoid them with the following codes after the product name:

> **G** – grapefruit seed extract
> **T** – titanium dioxide
> **Z** – zinc oxide

For for quick and easy reference, print a copy of these codes from www.dyingtolookgood.com

Where to Find Recommended Products

Many of the products listed here are not found in the typical department store, grocery store, or pharmacy. All can be found at one or more of the following places:

- On the Internet
- Natural Food Stores
- Health Food Stores
- Food Co-Ops
- Mail-Order Health Catalogs

There's contact information for every product included here at the end of the product listing.

If you're willing to shop online, you'll find that your biggest problem will be deciding which products to buy. If you're uncomfortable using a credit card online, use the internet to decide what you want, then call and place your order over the phone. If the company's products are sold in retail stores, you'll usually find that information on their website too.

You'll find that there's no shortage of healthy products to choose from if you know how to find them and where to shop.

Healthy Products

MAKEUP

Foundation

Aubrey Organics
Natural Translucent Base
Burt's Bees
Tinted Facial Moisturizer [T]
Dr. Hauschka
Cover Stick [TZ]
Translucent Make-up [T]
Earth's Beauty
Mineral Colours Original Foundation Powder
Mineral Colours Plus SPF 15 Foundation Powder [Z]
Eternal Beauty™ Natural Mineral Cosmetics
Loose Mineral Foundation Powders [TZ]
All Natural Face Cream
Miessence
Translucent Foundation (all) [GZ]
The Organic Make-Up Company
Foundation [T]

Face powders

Aubrey Organics
Natural Translucent Base
Silken Earth (all)
Burt's Bees
Vanishing Facial Powder Tissues [TZ]
Vanishing Facial Powder [TZ]
Earth's Beauty
Mineral Colours Original Foundation Powder
Mineral Colours Plus SPF 15 Foundation Powder [Z]
Eternal Beauty™ Natural Mineral Cosmetics
Mineral Setting Powder
Mineral Bronzer [T]

Miessence
Translucent powder
Bronzing Dust
The Organic Make-Up Company
Face Powder

Blushes

Aubrey Organics
Silken Earth (all)
Burt's Bees
Blushing Crèmes [T]
Earth's Beauty
Mineral Colours Blush
Loose Powder Blush
Ecco Bella
Flower Color Bronzer [Z]
Eternal Beauty™ Natural Mineral Cosmetics
Mineral Blush [T]
Mineral Bronzer [T]
Multi-Purpose Mineral Powders [T]
Miessence
Mineral Blush Powder (all)
Shimmer Cremes (all)
The Organic Make-Up Company
Blushing Powder
Zuzu Luxe
Blush [TZ]

Concealers

Burt's Bees
Concealing Crème [T]
Earth's Beauty
Under Eye Concealer [T]
Ecco Bella
Natural Cover-Up [T]
Miessence
Concealer [GZ]

Paul Penders
 "Nutritious Color" Cover-up Sticks [T]
The Organic Make-Up Company
 Concealer [T]

Lipsticks, Glosses and Lip Pencils

Affusion Skin Care
 Soothing Lip Balm [G]
Botanical Skin Works
 Vitamin E Lip Balm
 Lip Butter
Burt's Bees
 Lip Gloss
 Beeswax Lip Balm
 Lifeguard's Choice Lip Balm [T]
 Lip Pencils [T]
 Lip Shimmers [T]
 Lipsticks [T]
Dr. Haushka
 Lip Care Stick
 Lip Balm
 Lipstick [T]
Earth's Beauty
 Lip Nectar
 Lip Glaze
 Lip Gloss
 Lip Liner
Ecco Bella
 Good For You Gloss
 Flower Color Lipstick
Hemp Organics
 Lipstick
 Lip Liners [T]
Miessence
 Jaffa Lip Balm
 Lip Creme (all) [Z]
 Shimmer Crème (all)

Natures Brands
Herbal Choice Body Care Natural Lip Balm
Paul Penders
"Nutritious Color" Lip Colors [T]
Lip Gloss [T]
Sassy Suds
Petroleum Free Lip Balms
Simmons Natural Bodycare
Simmons Lip Balm [G]
Sunflower Soaps & Sundries
` Lip Balms
SuperLan
SuperLan Tube
Terra Naturals
Lip Silk
Terressentials
100% Organic White Chocolate Lip Protector
100% Organic Mint White Chocolate Lip Protector
100% Organic Orange White Chocolate Lip
Protector
100% Organic Key Lime White Chocolate Lip
Protector
The Organic Make-Up Company
Lip Gloss
Lipstick
Lip Balm
The Vital Image
Lip & Skin Balm
Young Living
Cinnamint Lip Balm
Zuzu Luxe
Lipstick [T]

Eye Make-Up

Burt's Bees
Eye Shadow [TZ]
Eyeliner & Eyebrow Pencil [TZ]
Earth's Beauty
Mineral Colours Eye Shadow
Mineral Colours Eye Liner
Eternal Beauty™ Natural Mineral Cosmetics
Multi-Purpose Mineral Powders [T]
Cream To Powder Brow Definer & Eyeliner [1]
Matte Mineral Eye Shadows [T]
Morrocco Method, Int'l
Creamy Eyeliner
The Organic Make-Up Company
Eyeshadow Regular
Cream Shimmer Eye Shadow
Eye Shadow Wet/Dry
Cream Eyeshadow Base
Zuzu Luxe
Eyeshadow [TZ]

Mascara

Beauty Wise Cosmetics
Full'N Natural Mascara
Dr. Hauschka
Mascara [T]
Paul Penders
"Nutritious Color" Mascaras [G]
Real Purity
Mascara
Zuzu Luxe
Mascara

Makeup Removal

Affusion Skin Care
> Glycerin and Rosewater Spritz

Aubrey Organics
> Herbessence Makeup Remover [G]

Dr. Hauschka
> Cleansing Cream
> Cleansing Milk

Natures Brands
> Herbal Choice Body Care Natural Facial Cleanser

Paul Penders
> Natural Make-up Remover [G]

Fragrances & Perfumes

Aubrey Organics
> Eau de Cologne (all)

Earth's Beauty
> True Aroma Parfum Oils

Ecco Bella
> Eau De Parfum

Natures Brands
> Herbal Choice Body Care Ladies Perfume Balm
> Herbal Choice Body Care Gents Cologne Balm

Simmons Natural Bodycare
> Amber Essence
> Patchouli Essence
> Rose Essence
> Sandal Essence

Victorie Inc, 100% All Natural Products
> Body Mist Sprays, Colognes and Essences

Young Living
> Abundance
> Harmony
> Joy
> Live with Passion
> Sensation
> White Angelica

HAIR CARE

Shampoos

Burt's Bees
> Rosemary Mint Shampoo Bar
> Herbal Treatment Shampoo

CWS
> Fruit & Herb Shampoo [G]

Dr. Hauschka
> Pure Shampoo

J.R. Liggett's
> Bar Shampoo
> Moisturizing Body Scrub
> Foam Face & Body Wash

Miessence
> Desert Flower Shampoo [G]
> Lemon Myrtle Shampoo [G]

Morrocco Method, Int'l
> Pine Shale Shampoo
> Apple Cider Vinegar Shampoo
> Sea Essence Shampoo
> Earth Essence Shampoo

Nature's Brands
> Herbal Choice Body Care Rosemary & Chamomile Shampoo
> Herbal Choice Body Care Sage & Thyme Natural Shampoo
> Herbal Choice Body Care Tea Tree Oil Natural Shampoo
> Herbal Choice Body Care Unscented Natural Shampoo

Paul Penders
> Walnut Oil Shampoo [G]
> Rosemary Shampoo [G]
> Jasmine Shampoo [G]

Real Purity
> Chamomile Shampoo

Native Earth Unscented Shampoo
Native Earth Scented Shampoo
Sea Chi Organics
Tasmanian Lavender Shampoo [G]
Terra Naturals
Hemp & Peppermint Shampoo
Neroli Blossom Shampoo
Shampoo Base
Tea Tree Shampoo & Body Wash
Terressentials
Pure Earth Hair Wash
The Vital Image
Hair Renewal Shampoo

Dandruff Shampoos & Conditioners

Natures Brands
Herbal-Medi-Care Natural Antifungal Dandruff
Shampoo
Herbal Choice Body Care Natural Conditioning
Rinse
Paul Penders
Pegaga Scalp Cleansing Treatment [G]
Holy Basil Conditioning Scalp Toner [G]

Conditioners

Aubrey Organics
Aloe Essence Shine Booster & Detangler
Jojoba & Aloe Desert Herb Revitalizing
Conditioner [G]
White Camellia Ultra Smoothing Conditioner [G]
Honeysuckle Rose Moisturizing Conditioner [G]
CWS
Herbal Conditioner [G]
Dr. Hauschka
Neem Hair Lotion

Living Nature
Manuka Nourishing Conditioner [G]
Miessence
Clarifying Citrus Rinse [G]
Protect B5 Hair Repair [G]
Shine Herbal Hair Conditioner [G]
Morrocco Method, Int'l
Diamond Crystal Mist Conditioner
Chi Instant Conditioner
Natures Brands
Herbal Choice Body Care Natural Conditioning Rinse
Organic Excellence
Mint Conditioner
Paul Penders
Lemon Perfecting Rinse [G]
Herbal Hair Repair Conditioning Treatment [G]
Real Purity
Citrus Hair Rinse
Native Earth Unscented Hair Rinse
Sea Chi Organics
Hair Growth Formula & Moisturizing Hair Treatment [G]
The Vital Image
Hair Therapy - Conditioner/Rinse

Women's Hair Coloring Products

Aubrey Organics
Color Me Natural
Light Mountain Henna
Henna Hair Color & Conditioner
Color the Gray Henna Hair Color & Conditioner
Morrocco Method, Int'l
Organic Henna: 100% Natural Hair Coloring

Hairsprays and Styling Products

Aubrey Organics
>Aloe Essence Organic Regular Hold Hairspray

Beauty Wise Cosmetics
>Natural Styling Spray [G]
>Natural Styling Gel [G]

Morrocco Method, Int'l
>Volumizer Mist Conditioner
>Blood of the Dragon Styling Gel

Natural Health Supply
>Natural Hair Spray

Organic Excellence
>Alcohol-Free Hair Spray [T]

Real Purity
>Herbal Hair Spray
>Herbal Sensitive Hair Spray

DENTAL & ORAL HYGIENE

Toothpastes & Powders

A. Vogel
>Echinacea Toothpaste

Burt's Bees
>Cinna Mint Toothpaste
>Lavender Mint Toothpaste

Miessence
>Mint Toothpaste [G]
>Lemon Toothpaste [G]
>Anise Toothpaste [G]

Natural Health Supply
>Oregano Spearmint Tooth Powder

Natures Brands
>Herbal Choice Body Care Peppermint Toothpaste
>Herbal Choice Body Care Fennel Toothpaste
>Herbal Choice Body Care Cinnamon Toothpaste
>Herbal Choice Body Care Clove Toothpaste (for sensitive teeth)

Peelu
>Meswak Herbal Toothpaste
>Peppermint Toothpaste [T]
>Cinnamon Toothpaste [T]
>Spearmint Toothpaste [T]
>Plain Toothpaste [T]

Weleda
>Calendula Toothpaste
>Pink Toothpaste with Ratanhia

Young Living
>Dentarome Toothpaste
>Dentarome Plus Toothpaste

An alternative to toothpaste is plain and simple baking soda.

Mouthwashes & Breath Fresheners

A. Vogel
>   Dentaforce Herbal Mouth Spray

Aubrey
>   Natural Mint Mouthwash

Burt's Bees
>   Peppermint Breath Drops

Miessence
>   Freshening Mouthwash [G]

Natures Brands
>   Herbal Choice Body Care Natural Mouth Wash

Terra Naturals
>   Mouthwash (Wakey Wakey)

Weleda
>   Ratanhia Mouthwash

Young Living
>   Fresh Essence Plus Mouthwash

FEMININE HYGIENE

Menstrual Products

Happy Heiny
>Cloth Reusable Menstrual Pads

Feminine Options
>Cotton Reusable Menstrual Pads
>The Diva Cup Menstrual Cup

Lunapads Natural Menstrual Products
>Lunapads
>Lunapanties
>Lunaliners

Natracare Personal Hygiene
>Organic Cotton Tampons
>- Regular
>- Super
>- Super Plus
>
>Disposable Pads and Liners
>Organic Cotton Disposable Wipes

Organic Essentials Hygiene Products
>Organic Cotton Tampons
>- Regular
>- Super

Pleasure Puss®
>Cloth Reusable Sanitary Pads

Sea Pearls
>Natural Sea Sponge Tampons

The Diva Cup
>Menstrual Cup

The Keeper
>Menstrual Cup

The Mooncup
>Menstrual Cup

SKIN PRODUCTS

Antiperspirants & Deodorants

Aubrey
Calendula Blossom Natural Deodorant Spray
E Plus High C Roll-On Deodorant
Burt's Bees
Herbal Deodorant
Common Sense Farm
Lady Fern Deodorant [G]
Vetiver & Spice Deodorant [G]
Dr. Haushka
Deodorant Floral
Deodorant Fresh
Lavera
Deodorant Spray
Miessence
Ancient Spice Deodorant [G]
Tahitian Breeze Deodorant [G]
Aroma-Free Deodorant [G]
Real Purity
Holistic Roll On Deodorant
Simmons Natural Bodycare
Deodorant Crystal
Terra Naturals
Floral Actives Deodorant Sticks
Crystal Salt Deodorant Stone
Deodorant Spray Mists
Himalayan Crystal Deodorant Salt Bars
Terressentials
Organic Fragrance-free Deodorant
Organic Zen Spice Deodorant
Organic Lavender Fresh Deodorant
Organic Zesty Citrus Deodorant
The Vital Image
Sea Breeze – Organic Body Freshener

True Aroma

Lavender & Citrus Deodorant Stick

Weleda

Citrus Deodorant

Young Living

Aromaguard [Z]

Bath Oils, Mineral Baths & Special Baths

Affusion Skin Care

Lavender Essential Oil

Bath and Massage Oil

Aubrey Organics

Natural Spa Sea Wonders Invigorating Bath Salts

Natural Spa Sea Wonders Relaxing Bath Salts

Camomile Calming Bath Soak

Relax-R-Bath Soothing Herbal Bath Emulsion [G]

Rosa Mosqueta® Moisturizing Bath & Shower Gel [G]

NSB (Natural Sports Bath) [G]

Botanical Skin Works

Bath Salts

Detox Bath Salts

Burt's Bees

Vitamin E Body & Bath Oil

Therapeutic Bath Crystals

Chi Herbal Infusions

Chi Harmonizing Bath [G]

Elysian Dream

Bath Salts

Milk Bath

Natures Brands

Herbal Choice Body Care Aromatherapy Bath Oil

Herbal Choice Body Care Aromatherapy Bath
Crystals

Sassy Suds

Bath Salts (uncolored)

Silk'N Shea

Bath & Body Oil

Simply Sea Salt

Salt Scrub
Silken Soles Soak
Silken Soles Scrub
Silken Soles Salts
Cleopatra's Foaming Milk Bath
Simmons Natural Bodycare
Mtn Rose Bath Herbs
Sunflower Soaps & Sundries
Bath Crystals
Bath Oils
Bath Teas
Terra Naturals
Bath Salts
Himalayan Crystal Bath Salts
Weleda
Citrus Refreshing Bath Milk
Lavender Relaxing Bath Milk
Pine Reviving Bath Milk
Rosemary Invigorating Bath Milk
Young Living
Aqua Essence Bath Pack
Bath Gel Base

Blemish Care Preparations

Affusion Skin Care
Tea Tree Essential Oil
Tea Tree and Rosemary Essential Oil
Aroma Bella
Acne Gel
Botanical Skin Works
Acne Treatment Gel
Burt's Bees
Herbal Blemish Stick
Miessence
Purifying Blemish Gel [G]
Natures Brands
Herbal Choice Body Care Facial Spot Treatment

Paul Penders
Blemish Away
Terra Naturals
Acne Gel

Facial Masks

Affusion Skin Care
Refreshing Clay Mask
Aroma Bella
Deep Pore Facial Masque
Moisturizing Lemin Grass Facial Masque
Stimulating Mint Facial Masque [Z]
Dr. Haushka
Facial Steam Bath
Cleansing Clay Mask
Rejuvenating Mask
Miessence
Mineral Mask (all)
Natures Brands
Herbal Choice Body Care Natural Facial Mask
Terra Naturals
Face Mask
Terressentials
100% Organic Flower Therapy Flower Acid Facial
Masque
The Organic Make-Up Company
Dead Sea Mud Mask
The Vital Image
Clay Masque

Massage Oils

Affusion Skin Care
Bath and Massage Oil
Aroma Bella
Body Oils (all)

Aubrey

Natural Spa Sea Wonders Invigorating Massage Oil
Natural Spa Sea Wonders Unscented Massage Lotion
Natural Spa Sea Wonders Relaxing Massage Oil

Blue Moon Herbals

Massage & Body Oils

Young Living

Cel-Lite Magic
Dragon Time Massage
Ortho Ease
Ortho Sport
Relaxation
Sensation Massage
V-6 Mixing Oil

Moisturizers

Aroma Bella

Ultra Rich Moisturizer
Ultra Light Moisturizer
Vitamin A Moisturizer
Plantagen Moisturizer
Plantagen Night Cream
Avonique Oil

Dr. Hauschka

Moisturizing Day Cream
Rose Body Moisturizer

Miessence

Moisturiser (all) [G]

Paul Penders

Hydrating Control Serum
St. Johns Wort Day Time Moisturizer [GT]
Wheatgerm Night Time Moisturizer [GT]
Aloe & Lavender Day Time Moisturizer [GT]
Avocado Night Time Moisturizer [GT]
Hibiscus Rose Day Time Moisturizer [GT]
Mangosteen Night Time Moisturizer [GT]

Terra Naturals
>Floral Actives Moisturizer
>Hydrating Lipids
>Floral Face Mist

Terressentials
>100% Organic Fragrance-free Moisture Cream

The Vital Image
>C-Serum + MSM
>Lipid Complex

Powders For Body Care

Botanical Skin Works
>Lavender Body Powder
>Herbal Foot Powder

Miessence
>Luxurious Body Powder

Sunflower Soaps & Sundries
>Dusting Powders

Shaving Creams

Affusion Skin Care
>Shaving Soap

Botanical Skin Works
>Bay Lime Shaving Gel
>Bay Lime Beard Conditioning Oil
>Bay Lime Soothing After Shave

Silk'N Shea
>Gentle After-Shave

Simmons Natural Bodycare
>Aloe Vera Shaving Soap

Skin Lotions, Creams and Toners

Affusion Skin Care
>Herbal Replenishing Cream [G]
>Day Cream with Zinc Oxide [Z]
>Glycerin and Rosewater Spritz

Lavender and Germanium Essential Oil
Toner for Normal to Dry Skin [G]
Toner for Normal to Oily Skin [G]

Aroma Bella
Moisturizing Body Lotion (all)
Aloe Toner Skin Soother
Aloe Astringent Skin Soother
Peppermint Foot Cream

Aubrey
Angelica Hand & Body Cream with White Camellia
Morning Musk Hand & Body Cream
Evening Primrose Soothing Hand & Body Lotion [G]
Sea Buckthorn with Ester-C® Nourishing Hand & Body Lotion [G]
Ultimate Moist Green Tea Rosemary Mint Hand & Body Lotion [G]
Ultimate Moist Passionflower Hand & Body Lotion [G]
Ultimate Moist Unscented Hand & Body Lotion [G]

Blue Moon Herbals
Crystal Essence Body Butters
Massage & Body Oils
Balms
Raw Shea Butter

Botanical Skin Works
Shea Butter Body Cream
Body Cream
Beautiful Body Butter
Whipped Body Butter
Unrefined Shea Butter
Cocoa Butter
Rose Bulgaria/Mint Spritz
Luxurious Hand Cream
Unscented Hand Cream
Herbal Foot Cream

Burt's Bees
Carrot Nutritive Body Lotion
Vitamin E Body & Bath Oil
Shea Buter Hand Repair Crème
Hand Salve

Chi Herbal Infusions
>Chi Herbal Harmonizing Spray [G]
>Chi Herbal Purifier [G]
>Chi Purifier Lotion [G]

Common Sense Farm
>Jojoba Rose Lotion
>Lemon Cypress Lotion
>Chamomile Primrose Lotion
>Shea Butter Lotion
>Shea Butter

Dr. Hauschka
>Facial Toner
>Clarifying toner
>Rhythmic Night Conditioner
>Rhythmic Conditioner, Sensitive
>Rose Day Cream
>Normalizing Day Oil
>Toned Day Cream [T]
>Eye Contour Day Balm
>Rosemary Foot Balm
>Quince Day Cream
>Translucent Bronze Concentrate Hand Cream
>St. John's Wort Foot Cream [7]

Ecco Bella
>Organic Facial Treatment Serums

Eternal Beauty™ Natural Mineral Cosmetics
>All Natural Face Cream

Miessence
>Skin Conditioner (all) [G]
>Intensive Body Cream [G]

Natural Innovations
>MSM Natural Lotion [G]
>Rainforest MSM Natural Lotion [G]
>MSM Natural Berry Vanilla Lotion [G]
>Emotion Lotion [G]
>Nature's Silk Goat's Milk Lotion [G]

Natures Brands
>Herbal Choice Body Care Hand & Body Lotion

Herbal Choice Body Care Aromatherapy After Bath Lotion

Herbal Choice Body Care Gentle Eye Cream

Herbal Choice Body Care Facial & Body Oil

Herbal Choice Body Care Natural Vitamin E Oil

Herbal Choice Body Care Natural Facial Toner

Paul Penders

Orangeblossom Skin Toner [G]

Chamomile Skin Toner [G]

Moringa Skin Toner [G]

Sea Chi Organics

Sea Chi Crème

Moroccan Blue Chamomile Body Oil

Tasmanian Lavender Body Oil

Sea Chi Certified Organic Jojoba Oil

Rose Water & Kombuchi Firming Facial Toner

Silk"N Shea

TLC Balm

Eye Cream

Silken Soles Salve

Simmons Natural Bodycare

Mtn Rose Wildcraft Cream

Aromalotion [G]

Cocoa Butter Crème [G]

Duck Butter [G]

Mtn Rose Powerful Skin Compound

SuperLan

SuperLan

SuperLan Lite Moisturizer

Terra Naturals

Chamomile Body Elixir

Orange Blossom Body Elixir

Lavender Body Elixir

Sage Foot Oil

Foot Care Treatment

Terressentials

Flower Therapy Daily Renewal Facial Lotion

Flower Therapy Replenishing Facial Cream

Flower Therapy Silken Velvet Body Lotion

Fragrance-free Organic Silken Velvet Body Lotion
100% Organic Anointing Body Oils
100% Organic Body Crème Push-ups
100% Organic Cocoa Butter Rich Body Oil
100% Organic Cocoa Butter Body Crème Push-up
100% Organic Pure Cocoa Butter Push-up

The Organic Make-Up Company
Athletic Body Butter
Face Cream
Hand Lotion
Alcohol-Free Face Toner

The Vital Image
Hand and Foot Cream
Shower Silk

Victorie Inc, 100% All Natural Products
Eternal Beauty all Natural Face Cream
Natural Hand & Body Lotion

Weleda
Birch Cellulite Oil
Citrus Body Oil
Foot Balm

Women's Therapeutic Institute
Progestelle

Young Living
Rose Ointment
Genesis Hand & Body Lotion
Sandalwood Toner
Satin Body Lotion
Sensation Hand & Body Lotion

Skin Rejuvenation

Aroma Bella
>Eye Repair Crème
>Sea Weed Gel
>Lifting Botanical Gel
>Topical Skin Supplement

Miessence
>Rejuvenessence Facial Serum
>Firming Eye & Neck Serum [G]
>Rose Monsoon Hydrating Mist [G]

Natures Brands
>Herbal Choice Body Care Heel & Foot Cream

Paul Penders
>ICT (Intensive Clarifying Therapy) [G]
>Hydrating Control Serum
>Aqualuna [GT]

Terra Naturals
>Wrinkle Guard

Terressentials
>Flower Therapy Daily Renewal Facial Lotion
>Flower Therapy Replenishing Facial Cream

The Organic Make-Up Company
>Facial Oils

The Vital Image
>Skin Renewal Complex [Z]
>Pumpkin Antioxidant Masque
>Amino Complex
>Pot of Gold Night Repair [Z]
>Eye Area Builder
>Bag Buster for Under-Eye Bags
>Nourishing Body Milk
>Cleopatra's Dream
>CollagenBuilder

Weleda
>Iris Facial Toner
>Iris Moisture Cream

Young Living

Lavaderm Cooling Mist

Boswelia Wrinkle Cream

Soaps, Scrubs and Skin Cleansers

Affusion Skin Care

Castile Soap with 100% Olive Oil

Tea Tree Liquid Soap [G]

Lavender and Germanium Liquid Soap

Hand and Body Scrub

Alchemy Soapworks

Castile Soap

Sensitive Skin Soap

Luxury Soap

Aroma Bella

Gentle Emulsion Skin Cleanser

Citrus Gel Skin Cleanser

Candy Mint Facial Scrub

10% Exfoliating Face Wash

15% Exfoliating Face Wash

10% Fruit Acids Serum

15% Fruit Acids Serum

10% Exfoliating Masque [G]

15% Exfoliating Masque [G]

Aubrey Organics

Rosa Mosqueta® Moisturizing Cleansing Bar

Evening Primrose & Lavender Skin Care Bar

Honeysuckle Rose® Vegetal Soap

Meal & Herbs Exfoliation Skin Care Bar

Sea Buckthorn Skin Care Bar with Sandalwood [G]

White Camellia and Jasmine Emollient Soap [G]

Calaguala Skin Treatment Bar [G]

Rosa Mosqueta® Moisturizing Bath & Shower Gel [G]

Natural Spa Sea Wonders Sea Soap Shower Wash [G]

Natural Spa Sea Wonders Invigorating Body Polish [G]

Natural Spa Sea Wonders Relaxing Body Polish [G]

A Wild Soap Bar

Handcrafted Soaps

Blue Moon Herbals
>Bath Brews

Botanical Skin Works
>Hand Crafted Soaps
>Liquid Hand Soap
>Herbal Foot Scrub
>Herbal Foot Wash
>Tropical Salt Scrub
>Bay Lime Shower Gel
>Bay Lime Body Bar

Burt's Bees
>Peppermint Shower Soap
>Citrus Spice Exfoliating Shower Soap

Chi Herbal Infusions
>Chi Harmonizing Mask [G]
>Chi Cleansing Scrub [G]
>Chi Purifier Gel [G]

Common Sense Farm
>Fresh Mint Body Scrub
>Sweet Berry Fruit Scrub
>Tropical Castile Bodywash [G]
>Peppermint Castile Bodywash [G]

CWS
>Bar Soaps
>Bar Goat Milk Soaps
>Aloe & Castile Liquid Soap
>Shower Gels

Dr. Hauschka
>Lavender Bath
>Lemon Bath
>Rosemary Bath
>Sage Bath
>Spruce Bath

Ecco Bella
>Big Bar Soaps

Elysian Dream
>SuperMild Liquid Soap
>Castile Soap Bar
>Castile Liquid Soap

Miessence
Sunshower Body Wash [G]
Cleanser (all) [G]
Exfoliant (all) [G]

Morrocco Method, Int'l
Celtic Sea Salt® Lavender Shea Scrub
Celtic Sea Salt® Bath Crystals
Lavender Celtic Sea Soap®
Rosemary/Lemon Celtic Sea Soap®

Naikid Soaps
Botanical Soap
Scentuous Soap
Unscented Soap
Pure Soap
Milk Soap
Gritty Soap
Massage Soap

Natural Health Supply
Olive Oil Liquid Soap
Olive Oil Vegetarian Oval Soap

Natures Brands
Herbal Choice Body Care Handmade Beauty Soap
Herbal Choice Body Care Natural Facial Scrub
Herbal Choice Body Care Natural Facial Wash
Herbal Choice Body Care Natural Body Wash
Herbal Choice Body Care Foot Scrub

Paul Penders
Citrus Fruit Exfoliant [G]
Rosemary Cleansing Milk [G]
Calendula Cleansing Milk [G]
Alpinia Cleansing Milk [G]

Sassy Suds
Bar Soaps
Exfoliating Sea Spa Bar

Sea Chi Organics
Rose Geranium Face and Body Wash [G]

Silk"N Shea
Extra Gentle Bar Soap

Simmons Natural Bodycare
>Oatmeal Soap
>Mountain Mint Soap
>Orange Spice Soap
>Forest Soap
>French Lavender Soap
>Milk & Honey Soap
>Aloe Vera/Kelp Soap
>Sweet Almond Oil Soap
>Apricot Poppy Soap
>Mtn Rose Facial Scrub

Sunflower Soaps & Sundries
>Handmade Bar Soaps
>Handmade Liquid Soaps
>Salt Scrubs

Terra Naturals
>Daily Facial Cleanser
>Tea Tree Shampoo & Body Wash

Terressentials
>Flower Therapy Detoxifying Facial Cleanser
>Flower Therapy Exfoliating Facial Toner
>Real Soap for Hands – Organic Lovin' Lavender Tea Tree
>Real Soap for Hands – Organic Zingin' Citrus Tea Tree
>Real Soap for Hands – Organic Jammin' Spice Tea Tree
>Lavender Garden Body Wash
>Cool Mint Body Wash
>Left Coast Lemon Body Wash
>Sultry Spice Body Wash
>Fragrance-Free Gentle Bath Gel
>Natural Unscented Glycerine Soaps

The Organic Make-Up Company
>Exfoliant Cleanser
>Face Cleanser
>Soaps

The Vital Image

Face and Body Wash
Grime Fighter
Waterless Cleanser Toner
Skin Oxygenator
Oily Skin Cleanser

Victorie Inc, 100% All Natural Products

All Natural Bath & Shower Gel, Body Wash, Liquid
Soap
Unscented Dead Sea Salts
Aromatic Dead Sea Salts

Voda

Natural Soaps

Weleda

Iris Cleansing Lotion

Young Living

Lemon Sandalwood Bar Soap
Melaleuca Geranium Bar Soap
Morning Start Bar Soap
Peppermint Cedarwood Bar Soap
Sacred Mountain Bar Soap
Thieves Bar Soap
Valor Bar Soap
Lavender Rosewood Bar Soap
Evening Peace Shower Gel
Morning Start Shower Gel
Sensation Bath & Shower Gel

NAIL PRODUCTS

For Healthier Nails

Botanical Skin Works
>Anti-Fungal Nail Nutrient
>Critical Cuticle Treatment
>One Minute Manicure

Burt's Bees
>Lemon Butter Cuticle Crème

Dr. Haushka
>Neem Nail Oil

Natures Brands
>Herbal-Medi-Care Anti Fungal Ointment
>Homeo-Care Nail & Cuticle Cream

Nail Polishes, Hardeners & Protectors

Botanical Skin Works
>Nail Nutrient

Firozé Nail & Skin Care Products
>Nail Enhancer Base Coat
>Silk Enhancer Base Coat
>Pyramid White
>Talisman Coral
>Sunset Pink
>Glossy Top Coat
>Nail Rejuvenating & Cuticle Cream
>All Natural Conditioning Nail Polish Remover

Sante Kosmetics
>Nail Polish Remover

Terra Naturals
>Nail Strengthener

I'm not a fan of nail polish, even those with healthy natural ingredients, because your nails are porous and need to breathe. If you must use nail polish, do so only occasionally.

Artificial nails are harmful to your health. See page 25.

OUTDOOR PRODUCTS

Sunscreens & Suntan Oils/Lotions

Some of the products listed here are not sunscreens. Sunscreens may interfere with the body's ability to produce vitamin D. For more information on sunscreens and safe sun exposure, see page 36. Take a few minutes to learn how to enjoy the sun responsibly and safely.

Aubrey
 After Sun Natural Tanning Maintenance [G]
Barnacle Cove
 Mexitan Tanning Oil [TZ]
 Mexitan Dark Tanning Oil
 Mexitan Chemical-Free Sunscreen [TZ]
 Mexitan Chemical-Free After Sun Moisturizer
Botanical Skin Works
 Summer Bronzing Oil
Dr. Hauschka
 Sunscreen Lotion SPF8 [T]
 Sunscreen Lotion SPF15 [T]
 Sunscreen Lotion SPF20 [T]
 After-Sun Lotion
Living Nature
 Wild Pansy & Zinc Sunscreen [TZ]
Young Living
 Sunsation Suntan Oil

Insect Repellants

Affusion Skin Care
 Insect Repellent
Barnacle Cove
 Florida Special DEET Free Repellent
Botanical Skin Works
 Botanical Bug Repellant
Burt's Bees
 Herbal Insect Repellant

Miessence
  Buzz Free Zone Personal Spray [G]
Natures Brands
  Herbs 2 Heal Insect (mosquito) Repellant
Terra Naturals
  Shoofly Spray

BABIES & CHILDREN

Shampoos

Elysian Dream
> Baby Wash/ Shampoo
> Pure Castile Baby Soap

Miessence
> Desert Flower Shampoo

Terra Naturals
> Calendula Baby Shampoo

Baby Powders

Botanical Skin Works
> Baby Powder

Burt's Bees
> Baby Bee Dusting Powder

Common Sense Farm
> Baby Powder

Simmons Natural Bodycare
> Mtn Rose Baby's Body Powder

Terra Naturals
> Baby Dust

Lotions & Creams

Botanical Skin Works
> Calendula Baby Lotion
> Baby Massage Oil
> Baby Bottom Ointment
> Mommy's Belly Balm

Burt's Bees
> Apricot Baby Oil
> Baby Bee Diaper Ointment [Z]

Common Sense Farm
> Baby Lotion
> Baby Cream [Z]

Elysian Dream

Baby Bottom Balm

Silk'N Shea

Baby Balm

Baby Lotion

Simmons Natural Bodycare

Mtn Rose Baby's Balm

SuperLan

SuperLan

Terra Naturals

Nourishing Baby oil

Terressentials

Organic Baby Body Lotion

Organic Baby Massage Oil

100% Organic Terrific Tush Treatment

Young Living

Kidscents Lotion

Kidscents Tender Tush

Weleda

Diaper-Care

Calendula Baby Oil

Calendula Baby Lotion

Soaps

Affusion Skin Care

Castile Soap with 100% Olive Oil

Tea Tree Liquid Soap [G]

A Wild Soap Bar

Wee Wild Baby Soap

Botanical Skin Works

Baby Lavender Bath

Burt's Bees

Baby Bee Buttermilk Soap

CWS

Lavender Baby Bar Goat Milk Soap

Elysian Dream

Baby Shampoo & Body Wash

Castile Soap Bar

Castile Liquid Soap
Terra Naturals
Honeysuckle Soap
Terressentials
Organic Baby Wash

Baths Products

Botanical Skin Works
Baby Lavender Bath
Burt's Bees
Baby Bee Buttermilk Bath Pint

Little Girls Play Cosmetics

Little Earth's Beauty
Girls' Play Makeup Set
Body Glitter

Toothpastes

Burt's Bees
Children's Toothpaste
Weleda
Children's Tooth Gel
Young Living
Kidscents Bubble Gum Flavor Toothpaste
Dentarome Toothpaste

Disposable Diapers

100% cotton cloth diapers are preferable to disposable diapers. They give you more control over what chemicals come in contact with your baby's delicate bottom. But if you need the convenience of disposable diapers, or just for occasional use, here are some of the more natural, healthier choices on the market.

Nature Boy and Girl Diapers
>   Disposable diapers, corn based material

Seventh Generation
>   Chlorine-free diapers

TenderCare
>   Chlorine Free Diapers

Tushies Disposable Diapers & Wipes
>   Diapers, Gel-Free

Wipes

A warm, wet, 100% cotton wash cloth with pure gentle soap is the best wipe for your baby's bottom. You can even carry them with you in a diaper bag. They're more cost effective in the long run too. But, if you have to have disposable wipes, these are the best ones I've found, but they do contain a little preservative.

Tushies Disposable Diapers & Wipes
>   TushiesWipes, Unscented
>   Mother Nature Flushable Wipes
>   Flushable TenderCare Wipes, Unscented

Sunscreen

Sunscreens may interfere with the body's ability to produce vitamin D. Before using sunscreen on your babies and children, read about sunscreens and safe sun exposure on page 36.

Barnacle Cove
>   Mexitan Chemical-Free Sunscreen SPF 30 for Kids [TZ]

Dr. Hauschka
>   Sunscreen Cream for Children SPF22 [T]

Insect Repellants

Affusion Skin Care
> Insect Repellent

Barnacle Cove
> Florida Special DEET Free Repellent:

Burt's Bees
> Herbal Insect Repellant

PET PRODUCTS

Aubrey
> Organimals Grooming Spray For Dogs [G]
> Organimals Dip & Crème Rinse Concentrate For Dogs [G]

Earthy Pet
> Pet Shampoo – Flea Relief Formula

Young Living
> Animal Scents Pet Ointment
> Animal Scents Pet Shampoo

RESOURCES – WHERE TO BUY

Affusion Skin Care
affusionskincare.dyingtolookgood.com
877-842-8120
770-664-0096

Alchemy Soapworks
alchemysoapworks.dyingtolookgood.com
770-466-9950

All Natural Cosmetics
allnaturalcosmetics.dyingtolookgood.com
888-586-9719
928-772-0119
> Common Sense Farm
> CWS
> Earth's Beauty
> Earthy Pet
> Hemp Organics
> Lavera
> Light Mountain Henna
> Living Nature
> Miessence
> Organic Excellence
> Real Purity
> True Aroma

Aroma Bella
aromabella.dyingtolookgood.com
800-760-7779
843-559-7541

Aubrey Organics
aubrey-organics.dyingtolookgood.com
800-282-7394

A. Vogel
bioforce.dyingtolookgood.com
800-361-6320

A Wild Soap Bar
awildsoapbar.dyingtolookgood.com
512-272-4058

Baby's Bottom Line
babysbottomline.dyingtolookgood.com
206-301-9456
> Nature Boy and Girl Diapers
> TenderCare Chlorine Free Diapers
> Tushies Diapers

Barnacle Cove
Mexitan
mexitan.dyingtolookgood.com
239-947-1327

Beauty Wise Cosmetics
holisticbeauty.dyingtolookgood.com
bewellstaywell.dyingtolookgood.com

Blue Moon Herbals
bluemoonherbals.dyingtolookgood.com
732-793-6656
877-596-1772

Botanical Skin Works
botanicalworks.dyingtolookgood.com
410-675-2006

Burt's Bees
burtsbees.dyingtolookgood.com

Chi Herbal Infusions
chiformulas.dyingtolookgood.com
619-309-9418

Common Sense Farm
commonsensefarm.dyingtolookgood.com
518-677-0224
allnaturalcosmetics.dyingtolookgood.com

CWS
allnaturalcosmetics.dyingtolookgood.com

Dr. Hauschka
drhauschka.dyingtolookgood.com
800-247-9907

Earth's Beauty
earthsbeauty.dyingtolookgood.com
888-586-9719
928-772-0119

Earthy Pet
allnaturalcosmetics.dyingtolookgood.com

Ecco Bella
eccobella.dyingtolookgood.com
877-696-2220
973-655-9585

Elysian Dream
elysiandream.dyingtolookgood.com

Eternal Beauty™ Natural Mineral Cosmetics
Victorie Inc, 100% All Natural Products
eternalbeauty.dyingtolookgood.com
866-457-3824

Feminine Options
feminineoptions.dyingtolookgood.com
614-477-1567
       Diva Cup
       Cotton Menstrual Pads

Firozé Nail & Skin Care Products
firoze.dyingtolookgood.com
866-866-1316
860-355-5214

Happy Heiny Cloth Menstrual Pads
jacksmagicbeanstalk.dyingtolookgood.com

Hemp Organics
allnaturalcosmetics.dyingtolookgood.com
veganessentials.dyingtolookgood.com

Holistic Beauty
holisticbeauty.dyingtolookgood.com
877-232-5359
330-337-0703
         Beauty Wise Cosmetics
         Living Nature
         Real Purity

Jack's Magic Beanstalk
jacksmagicbeanstalk.dyingtolookgood.com
1-877-7363
         Happy Heine Menstrual Pads
         Natural Parenting Store

J.R. Liggett's
jrliggett.dyingtolookgood.com
603-675-2055

Lavera
allnaturalcosmetics.dyingtolookgood.com

Light Mountain Henna
allnaturalcosmetics.dyingtolookgood.com

Little Earth's Beauty
allnaturalcosmetics.dyingtolookgood.com

Living Nature
livingnature.dyingtolookgood.com
+64 9 4077895
allnaturalcosmetics.dyingtolookgood.com

Lunapads International Products Ltd.
lunapads.dyingtolookgood.com
888-590-2299

Miessence
miessence.dyingtolookgood.com
allnaturalcosmetics.dyingtolookgood.com

Morrocco Method, Int'l
morroccomethod.dyingtolookgood.com
805-534-1600

Naikid Soaps
naikid.dyingtolookgood.com

Natracare Personal Hygiene
shopnatural.dyingtolookgood.com

Natural Health Supply
naturalhealthsupply.dyingtolookgood.com
866-355-1272

Natural Innovations Nutrition, Inc.
Available through healthcare professionals
888-719-8998

NaturalSolutions
Holistic Beauty, Body & Bath
bewellstaywell.dyingtolookgood.com
877-232-5359
330-337-0703
        Organic Makeup Co.
        Living Nature
        Real Purity

Beauty Wise Cosmetics
Sante Cosmetics

Nature Boy and Girl Diapers
babysbottomline.dyingtolookgood.com

Natures Brands
NaturallyDirect.net
naturesbrands.dyingtolookgood.com
888-417-1375
570-223-6724
Herbal Choice Body Care
Herbal-Medi-Care
Herbs 2 Heal
Homeo-Care

Organic Essentials Hygiene Products
shopnatural.dyingtolookgood.com

Organic Excellence
allnaturalcosmetics.dyingtolookgood.com

Paul Penders
paulpenders.dyingtolookgood.com

Peelu
shopnatural.dyingtolookgood.com

Pleasure Puss Cloth Pads
pleasurepussclothpads.dyingtolookgood.com
61 2 66723065

Real Purity
realpurity.dyingtolookgood.com
931-788-5332
800-253-1694
allnaturalcosmetics.dyingtolookgood.com

Sante Kosmetics
holisticbeauty.dyingtolookgood.com

Sassy Suds
sassysuds.dyingtolookgood.com
877-277-7627

Sea Chi Organics
seachi.dyingtolookgood.com

Sea Pearls
shopnatural.dyingtolookgood.com

Seventh Generation
shopnatural.dyingtolookgood.com

ShopNatural™
shopnatural.dyingtolookgood.com
520-884-0745
> Burt's Bees
> Natracare
> Organic Essentials
> Peelu Toothpaste
> Sea Pearls
> Seventh Generation
> Tushies Disposable Diapers and Wipes

Silk'n Shea
silknshea.dyingtolookgood.com
503-244-2193

Simmons Natural Bodycare
simmonsnaturals.dyingtolookgood.com
707-777-1920

Sunflower Soaps & Sundries
sunflowersoapsandsundries.dyingtolookgood.com
760-294-1405

SuperLan
superlanolin.dyingtolookgood.com
845-352-7331

TenderCare Chlorine Free Diapers
babysbottomline.dyingtolookgood.com

Terra Naturals
terranaturals.dyingtolookgood.com
416-907-2483

Terressentials
terressentials.dyingtolookgood.com
301 371-7333

The Diva Cup
divacup.dyingtolookgood.com

The Keeper
thekeeper.dyingtolookgood.com
1-800-500-0077

The Mooncup
themooncup.dyingtolookgood.com
01273 673845

The Organic Make-Up Company
theorganicmakeupco.dyingtolookgood.com
905-479-9295

The Vital Image
thevitalimage.dyingtolookgood.com
800-414-4624
310-823-1996

True Aroma
allnaturalcosmetics.dyingtolookgood.com
earthsbeauty.dyingtolookgood.com

Tushies Disposable Diapers & Wipes
tushies.dyingtolookgood.com
shopnatural.dyingtolookgood.com

VeganEssentials.com
veganessentials.dyingtolookgood.com
866-88-VEGAN
414-527-9684
Ecco Bella
Hemp Organics
Paul Penders
Zuzu Luxe

Victorie Inc, 100% All Natural Products
Biblical Botanicals™
victorie.dyingtolookgood.com
866-457-3824

Voda
vodasoap.dyingtolookgood.com
203-364-8612

Weleda
weleda.dyingtolookgood.com
800-241-1030

Women's Therapeutic Institute
womhoo.dyingtolookgood.com
719-687-3438

Young Living
youngliving.dyingtolookgood.com

Zuzu Luxe
veganessentials.dyingtolookgood.com

Additional Resources for Finding Safer Products

Guide to Less Toxic Products
www.lesstoxicguide.ca
Produced by the Environmental Health Association of Nova
Scotia

Environmental Working Group (EWG)
www.ewg.org/reports/skindeep
Safety Assessment of Ingredients in Personal Care Products

Compares the ingredients in 7500 personal care products with
lists of chemicals used in the cosmetics industry:
- known to have health risks
- not tested for safety

Stay Up-To-Date On the Latest Information

This is a dynamic field. There's new technology, new
ingredients and new companies and products coming into the
"healthy products" arena all the time. Manufacturers are
creative in their packaging and describing their products
because they know consumers are becoming more concerned
about healthy ingredients. Sometimes it can be extremely
difficult to determine if a product is healthy because the
package may withhold information about the product or its
ingredients or may misrepresent the contents inside.

To help you stay up-to-date on healthy products and the
ingredients in your personal care products, I've created
DyingToLookGood.com. You can come here to get updates,
new information, ask questions and find special discounts on
healthy products. You can also let me know about healthy
products you find that you think belong on the healthy
products list.

Sign up at www.dyingtolookgood.com to be notified when
new information is posted on DyingToLookGood.com.

Glossary

Allergen – may cause allergic or hypersensitivity reaction.

Antibacterial –destroys bacteria or suppresses their growth; used in treating infections, preserving food and cosmetics.

Antidandruff – prevents excess dandruff formation.

Anti-inflammatory – suppresses inflammation; reduces pain, heat, redness and swelling resulting from injury or infection.

Antimicrobial – kills microorganisms or suppresses their growth; used in preserving food and cosmetics.

Antioxidant – prevents oxidation, protects against free radicals and slows cell and tissue damage.

Astringent – causes the tissues to contract.

Carcinogen – causes cancer.

Carrier oil – oil used to dilute pure essential oils.

Cheilitis – inflammation of the lips.

CIR – Cosmetic Ingredient Review, an independent panel established by the Cosmetic, Toiletry and Fragrance Association (CTFA) in 1976 to review and assess the safety of ingredients used in cosmetics.

Colorant – color additive

Co-carcinogen – not a carcinogen by itself but can potentiate cancer when acting with carcinogenic agents.

Contact dermatitis – skin reaction that occurs after exposure to a substance that either irritates your skin or causes an allergic response.

Contact sensitization – a delayed allergic reaction resulting in allergic contact dermatitis.

Dermatitis – inflammation of the skin.

Essence – scent; solution of a volatile oil in alcohol.

Essential oil – natural, aromatic oils distilled from plants; volatile oils.

FDA approved colorant – color additives that the FDA has approved for use in food and cosmetics.

GRAS (Generally Recognized As Safe) – food additives that were in use before 1958 and were considered safe, even if they had never been tested; between 1958 and 1997, manufacturers had to submit a petition to the FDA for approval of a new food additive; in 1997, the FDA decided to let the manufacturers decide if an additive is GRAS and no longer required pre-market approval.

Herbs – plants, including leaves, bark, berries, roots, gums, seeds, stems and flowers that have been used for thousands of years to help maintain good health; may use harmful chemicals to extract the herbs or may use the herbs in concentrations too low to be of benefit; may cause adverse reactions or may be very beneficial.

Humectant – a substance which moistens or dilutes.

Hydrocarbon – an organic compound which contains only hydrogen and carbon, like coal, petroleum and natural gas; hydrocarbons used in cosmetics include, paraffin wax, mineral oil, petrolatum.

Irritant – causes irritation.

Mutagen – causes genetic changes and may lead to cancer or hereditary diseases.

Natural emollient – softening or soothing substance derived from natural sources.

Natural emulsifier – a substance derived from natural sources which causes oil and water to mix and form a stable mixture.

Natural preservatives – protect against the growth of microorganisms which cause spoilage in food and cosmetics, but have a limited shelf life compared to chemical preservatives which are added in large enough quantities to yield a 2 – 3 year shelf life.

Neurotoxic – poisonous or destructive to nerve tissue.

Neurotoxin – a substance that is poisonous or destructive to nerve tissue.

Nitrosating agents – chemical compounds classified as secondary amines, including DEA, MEA, TEA, that combine with nitrogen-containing compounds to form nitrosamines.

Nitrosamines – chemical compounds formed when secondary amines combine with nitrites. Most nitrosamines are carcinogenic.

Oleochemicals – derived from animal fats and vegetable oils, like palm oil, palm kernel oil and inedible tallow, to make fatty acid esters, fatty alcohols, fatty amines and fatty amides; trans fats; they are processed at high heat with toxic metals and petrochemicals; may contain harmful or cancer-causing contaminants, or cause allergic reactions; used in detergents, soaps and cosmetics.

OSHA – Occupational Safety & Health Administration in the US Department of Labor.

Penetration enhancer – increases absorption through the skin.

Petrochemicals – derived from petroleum or natural gas.

Photosensitivity – increased reaction of the skin to sunlight; may burn more easily; when using ingredients that cause photosensitivity, avoid direct sunlight for up to 12 hours.

Phototoxic chemical – harmless chemical, synthetic or natural, used in sunscreens which becomes toxic and causes adverse reactions due to biochemical reaction with UV rays of the sun

Phototoxicity – being phototoxic.

Preservatives – protect against the growth of microorganisms which cause spoilage in food and cosmetics.

Sensitizer – causes the body to react more strongly to a substance.

Sunscreen – protects against some or all of the harmful rays of the sun.

Surfactants – water soluble compounds that lower the surface tension of water allowing it to spread more easily; soaps, emulsifying agents; can be derived from "natural" sources, i.e. animal fats or vegetable oils, or from synthetic sources, i.e. petroleum; all surfactants are synthetic, whether derived from natural or synthetic sources because they are highly processed, distilled, fractionated and hydrogenated.

Synthetic emollient – softening or soothing substance derived from synthetic chemicals; most cause adverse skin reactions.

Synthetic emulsifier – a substance derived from synthetic chemicals that causes oil and water to mix and form a stable mixture; most cause adverse reactions.

Synthetic humectant – synthetic moisturizers; many cause adverse reactions.

Teratogen – causes birth defects.
Vitamin – a substance naturally occurring in food that is necessary for normal metabolic functioning of the body.
Xenoestrogens – chemicals that mimic estrogen in the body. They are also called endocrine disrupters. They are stored in body fat and block hormones from performing their normal functions. Some of the ways you can accumulate xenoestrogens in your body are from drinking water or beverages from plastic bottles, wrapping food in plastic wrap, storing or microwaving food in plastic containers, using laundry detergent, cosmetics or personal care products containing these chemicals, or from pesticides on your food. Xenoestrogens are credited with children reaching puberty earlier and earlier, and are suspected to be a factor in breast cancer.

REFERENCES

"1. Read 2. Rinse 3. Repeat: What You Need To Know About The Products You Use Every Day," The Ottawa Citizen, April 23, 2005.

"11th Report on Carcinogens, National Toxicology Program," ntp.niehs.nih.gov/index.cfm?objectid=32BA9724-F1F6-975E-7FCE50709CB4C932

Allan, Susan, "All Natural, Pure Organic, 100-Per-Cent Mayhem," The Ottawa Citizen; April 21, 2005.

Allan, Susan and Page, Shelley, "Bather Beware: What You Need To Know Before Buying Hair Dye, Baby Wash, AHAs And Organic Products," The Ottawa Citizen; April 23, 2005.

Allan, Susan, "The Baby in the Bathwater;" The Ottawa Citizen, April 19, 2005.

Allan, Susan, "You Are What You Eat ... Breathe ... Scrub ... Lather ... Spray," The Ottawa Citizen; April 22, 2005.

Antczak, Dr. Stephen and Gina, Cosmetics Unmasked. London: Thorsons, 2001.

"Are Cosmetic Products With Alpha Hydroxy Acids Safe?" www.4woman.gov/faq/cosmetics.htm#11

Blake, et.al. "Application of the Photocatalytic Chemistry of TiO2 to Disinfection and the Killing of Cancer Cells," Separation and Purification Methods; Vol 28 (1) 1999 p.1-50

Botanical Dermatology Database, bodd. cf.ac.uk

Breakthrough Updates You Need to Know on Vitamin D, www.mercola.com/2002/feb/23/vitamin_d.htm

Britton, Jade & Tamara Kircher, The Complete Book of Home Herbal Remedies. Buffalo, New York: Firefly Books, 1998.

Bunney, Sarah, Editor, The Illustrated Book of Herbs; Their Medicinal and Culinary Uses. New York: Gallery Books, 1984.

Castleman, Michael, The Healing Herbs. Emmaus, PA: Rodale Press, 1991.

Center for Science in the Public Interest, www.cspinet.org

Chevallier, Andrew, The Encyclopedia of Medicinal Plants. New York: DK Publishing, Inc., 1996.

Cho S-W, Seo I-W, Choi J-D, Joo I-S, "Inhibitory Effects Of Grapefruit Seed Extract (DF-100) On Growth And Toxin Production Of Penicillium Islandicum," J Korean Agric Chem Soc; 33 (2). 1990. 169-173. [Korean]

CIR High Priority Review List, www.cir-safety.org/priorities.shtml

"Click Here: ... For More About Chemicals, Cosmetics And Campaigns," The Ottawa Citizen; April 23, 2005.

Cosmetic Ingredient Hotlist - May 2005, www.hc-sc.gc.ca/hecs-sesc/cosmetics/hotlist_a-c.htm

Cosmetic Ingredient Review, www.cir-safety.org

"Cosmetic Ingredients: Understanding the Puffery," www.fda.gov/fdac/reprints/puffery.html

"Cosmetic Labeling," www.cfsan.fda.gov/~dms/cos-labl.html

Cosmetic, Toiletry and Fragrance Association, www.ctfa.org

"Cosmetics 101: What's Known -- And Not Known -- About Chemicals in Beauty Products," The Ottawa Citizen; April 23, 2005.

"Cosmetics and Your Health,"
www.4woman.gov/faq/cosmetics.htm#11

CTFA International Buyers' Guide, www.ctfa-buyersguide.org
Dorland's Illustrated Medical Dictionary

Eckhart, Peter, M.D., "Avoid Estrogenic Chemicals (Xenoestrogens),"
www.womhoo.com/index.asp?PageAction=Custom&ID=4

Eckhart, Peter, M.D., www.womhoo.com

"Endocrine Disrupting Chemicals,"
e.hormone.tulane.edu/edc.html

Environmental Working Group (EWG),
www.ewg.org/reports/skindeep

Environmental Working Group (EWG), "Safety Recommendations Ignored,"
http://www.ewg.org/reports/skindeep/report/safety_violations.php

Environmental Working Group (EWG), "Unassessed Ingredients,"
www.ewg.org/reports/skindeep/report/unstudied_ingredients.php

"Evaluation," www-cie.iarc.fr/monoeval/eval.html

"Exposure," www.terressentials.com/exposure.html

"Face Facts: A Common-Sense Guide To Chemicals And Cosmetics," The Ottawa Citizen; April 23, 2005.

"Face Facts: What You Need To Know About Chemicals You Use Every Day," The Ottawa Citizen; April 16, 2005.

Fallon, Sally, Nourishing Traditions. New Trends Publishing, 2001.

Farlow, Christine H., DC, Food Additives: A Shopper's Guide To What's Safe & What's Not. KISS For Health Publishing, 2004.

Farlow, Christine H., DC, Healthy Eating: For Extremely Busy People Who Don't Have Time For It. KISS For Health Publishing, 1998.

Farlow, Christine H., D.C., MSG Safety Report.

"FAQ's: Grapefruit Seed Extract," www.gfex.com/faq.htm

FDA Alerts Consumers About Adverse Events Associated With "Permanent Makeup," www.fda.gov/bbs/topics/ANSWERS/2004/ANS01295.html; July 2, 2004.

FDA Center for Food Safety & Applied Nutrition, vm.cfsan.fda.gov/

Fiorentin L ; Barioni Junior W, "Growth Inhibiton Moulds Of The Group Aspergillus Flavus By Grapefruit Seed Extract," Arq Bras Med Vet Zootec; 43 (3). 1991. 227-240. [Portuguese]

Gardiner, Anthony, Medicinal Herbs and Essential Oils. Edison, New Jersey: Chartwell Books, Inc., 1995.

Glaser, Aviva, "Ubiquitous Triclosan: A Common Antibacterial Agent Exposed" www.beyondpesticides.org/pesticides/factsheets/Triclosan%20cited.pdf

Grieve, M., A Modern Herbal. New York: Dover Publications, Inc., 1971. Volumes I and II.

"Guide to Less Toxic Products;" Environmental Health Association of Nova Scotia, www.lesstoxicguide.ca/index.asp?fetch=personal

"Hair Dye Dilemmas," www.cfsan.fda.gov/~dms/cos-818.html

Hampton, Aubrey, Natural Organic Hair and Skin Care. Tampa, Florida: Organica Press, 1987.

Hampton, Aubrey, What's in Your Cosmetics? Tucson, AZ: Odonian Press, 1995.

"Hidden Sources of Processed Free Glutamic Acid (MSG)," truthinlabeling.org/hiddensources.html

Higley, Connie and Alan, Reference Guide for Essential Oils. Olathe, KS: Abundant Health, 1998.

"How Safe Is Permanent Makeup?" my.webmd.com/content/article/89/100191.htm

"IARC Monographs on the Evaluation of Carcinogenic Risks to Humans," www-cie.iarc.fr

Kamazawa, et.al. "Effects of Titanium Ions and Particles on Neutrophil Function and Morphology." Biomaterials 2002 Sep 23 (17): 3757-64

Krauss, Beatrice H., Native Plants Used As Medicine in Hawaii.

Lewis, Grace Ross, 1001 Chemicals in Everyday Products, New York: John Wiley & Sons, Inc., 1999.

"Lists of IARC Evaluations" www-cie.iarc.fr/monoeval/grlist.html

Michalun, Natalia, Milady's Skin Care & Cosmetic Ingredients Dictionary, Second Edition. Albany, NY: Delmar, 2001.

Nonprescription Products: Formulations & Features '96-97. Washington, DC: American Pharmaceutical Association, 1996.

Ody, Penelope, The Complete Medicinal Herbal. New York: Dorling Kindersley, Inc., 1993.

Online Medical Dictionary, www.gralab.ac.uk

Page, Shelley, "Shades of Risk," The Ottawa Citizen, April 18, 2005.

Page, Shelley, "The Wrinkle in the Anti-Wrinkle Cream," The Ottawa Citizen, April 20, 2005.

Page, Shelley, "Think Before You Pink," The Ottawa Citizen, April 17, 2005.

Page, Shelley and Allan, Susan, "Not So Pretty: Most beauty routines include the use of carcinogens, allergens and other harmful substances," The Ottawa Citizen, April 16, 2005.

Page, Shelley and Allan, Susan, "The Great Cosmetics Debate," The Ottawa Citizen, April 16, 2005.

"Preamble to the IARC Monographs" www-cie.iarc.fr/monoeval/preamble.html

"Premier Ink Shades Associated with Adverse Reactions," www.cfsan.fda.gov/~dms/cos-tat2.html

Rajapakse, N, E Silva and A Kortenkamp. 2002, "Combining Xenoestrogens at Levels below Individual No-Observed-Effect Concentrations Dramatically Enhances Steroid Hormone Action," Environmental Health Perspectives 110:917-921, www.ourstolenfuture.org/NewScience/synergy/2002-08rajapakseetal.htm

Ryman, Daniele, Aromatherapy; The Complete Guide to Plant and Flower Essences for Health and Beauty. New York: Bantam Books, 1993.

"Saving Face: Cosmetic safety from 1 to 40," The Ottawa Citizen, April 23, 2005.

Schiller, Carol & David, Aromatherapy Oils: A Complete Guide. New York: Sterling Publishing Co., Inc., 1996.

Sharamon, Shalila and Bodo J. Baginski, The Healing Power of Grapefruit Seed. Lotus Light Publications, 1997.

Smeh, Nikolaus J., MS, Health Risks in Today's Cosmetics: The Handbook for a Lifetime of Healthy Skin and Hair. Alliance Publishing Co., 1994.

Spangler, Luita D., "Xenoestrogens and Breast Cancer: Nowhere to Run," www.fwhc.org/health/xeno.htm

Stabile, Toni, Everything You Want to Know About Cosmetics. New York: Dodd, Mead & Company, 1984.

Steinman, David & Samuel S. Epstein, M.D., The Safe Shopper's Bible: A Consumer's Guide to Nontoxic Household Products, Cosmetics and Food. New York: Macmillan, 1995.

Stewart, David, Ph.D., D.N.M., The Chemistry of Essential Oils Made Simple. CARE Publications, Marble Hill, MO, 2005.

Stryker, Lori B.Sc., B.H.Ec., B.Ed., "Titanium Dioxide: Toxic or Safe?"
www.organicmakeup.ca/CA/titaniumdioxide.asp

"Sunblock Can Actually Increase Your Cancer Risk,"
www.mercola.com/2003/jul/2/sunblock_cancer.htm

"Sunblock Does Not Stop Skin Cancer,"
www.mercola.com/2003/oct/18/sunblock_cancer.htm

Sundheim G, Langsrud S, "Natural And Acquired Resistance Of Bacteria Associated With Food Processing Environments To Disinfectant Containing An Extract From Grapefruit Seeds," Symposium Of The Society Of Applied Bacteriology And The Biodeterioration Society, Guildford, England, UK, April 23-24, 1995. International Biodeterioration & Biodegradation; 36 (3-4). 1995. 441-448.

"Sunlight Actually Prevents Cancer,"
www.mercola.com/2002/apr/3/sun_prevents_cancer.htm

"Tattoos and Permanent Makeup,"
www.cfsan.fda.gov/~dms/cos-204.html

Tenney, Louise, M.H., Today's Herbal Health, Third Edition. Prove, Utah: Woodland Books, 1992.

"The Dirt on Antibacterial Soaps,"
www.healthatoz.com/healthatoz/Atoz/hl/sp/home/alert091920
00.jsp

"The Healthy Person's Guide to Personal Care Ingredients,"
www.terressentials.com/ingredientguide.html

The National Organic Program, Definitions—Regulatory Text,
www.ams.usda.gov/nop/NOP/standards/DefineReg.html

The National Research Council,
www.nationalacademies.org/nrc

"The Truth About Oleochemicals,"
www.terressentials.com/truthaboutoleochemicals.html

"The Truth About Grapefruit Seed Extract,"
http://www.terressentials.com/truthaboutgse.html

"The Truth About Sunscreens & Personal Care Products,"
Organic Consumers Association,
www.organicconsumers.org/bodycare/sunscreen.cfm

Tierra, Michael, C.A., N.D., Planetary Herbology. Santa Fe,
New Mexico: Lotus Press, 1988.

"Titanium dioxide," Julie Maltby, Millenium Chemicals,
www.pra.org.uk/research/nanotechnology.htm

"Titanium dioxide," www.answers.com/topic/titanium-
dioxide

"Titanium-Oxide Photocatalyst," Three Bond Technical
News, January 1, 2004,
www.threebond.co.jp/en/technical/technicalnews/pdf/tech62.
pdf

"Trash Your Sunscreen and Other Summer Sun Tips,"
www.mercola.com/2004/may/26/summer_sun.htm

Truth in Labeling Campaign, www.truthinlabeling.org

Vance, Judi, Beauty to Die For. Lincoln, NE: toExcel Press,
2000.

Von Woedtke T ; Schluter B ; Pflegel P ; Lindequist U ;
Julich WD, "Aspects of the antimicrobial efficacy of
grapefruit seed extract and its relation to preservative

substances contained," Pharmazie; VOL 54 ISS Jun 1999, P452-456.

Vitamins.com, www.vitamins.com/encyclopedia

"Voices In The Great Cosmetics Debate," The Ottawa Citizen, April 23, 2005.

Von Woedtke T, Schluter B, Pflegel P, Lindequist U, Julich WD, "Aspects of the antimicrobial efficacy of grapefruit seed extract and its relation to preservative substances contained," Institute of Pharmacy, Ernst Moritz Arndt University, Greifswald, Germany, www.ncbi.nlm.nih.gov/entrez/query.fcgi?cmd=Retrieve&db=PubMed&list_uids=10399191&dopt=Abstract

West, Bruce, D.C., Health Alert Newsletter

"What Precautions Should I Follow When Using AHA Products?" www.4woman.gov/faq/cosmetics.htm#11

"Where is MSG hidden?" truthinlabeling.org/II.WhereIsMSG.html

Wilson, Roberta, The Complete Guide to Understanding & Using Aromatherapy for Vibrant Health & Beauty. New York: Avery Publishing Group, 1995.

Winter, Ruth, A Consumer's Dictionary of Cosmetic Ingredients. New York: Three Rivers Press, 1999.

Updates

DyingToLookGood.com is your resource for

- A printable list of the ingredient codes and product codes. You'll have the codes handy for quick and easy reference, no matter what page you're on.
- Getting updates. Get new information that's not in the book. Stay up-to-date with developments concerning cosmetics and personal care products on the market.
- Asking questions. Submit your questions and get answers from an expert.
- Articles. You'll find informative articles on topics relevant to cosmetics and personal care products, their ingredients and their safety.
- Links to healthy products. Only products that meet the Dying to Look Good safety standards will be listed on this site. So you can be sure that if you shop from this site you will be directed to safe and healthy products.
- Getting special discounts on healthy products. Every month there will be a featured product offered at a special discount to dyingtolookgood.com members.
- And more.

DyingToLookGood.com is your resource for new information not in the book. It will not duplicate information in the book.

Sign up at www.dyingtolookgood.com today. Membership is free for a limited time.

Books By This Author

DYING TO LOOK GOOD: The Disturbing Truth About What's Really in Your Cosmetics, Toiletries and Personal Care Products (2006, Second Edition, Completely Revised)
$12.95 + $4.50 S&H + 7.75% tax (CA residents)

FOOD ADDITIVES: A Shopper's Guide To What's Safe & What's Not (2004 Revised Edition)
$4.95 + $1.75 S&H + 7.75% tax (CA residents)

HEALTHY EATING: For Extremely Busy People Who Don't Have Time For It.
$7.95 + $3.00 S&H + 7.75% tax (CA residents)

When ordering more than one book, call or e-mail for S&H charges.

To order, send check or money order to:

KISS For Health Publishing
P.O. Box 462335-C
Escondido, CA 92046-2335
(760) 735-8101
e-mail: kiss4health@lycos.com

Excerpts, information on the contents of these books and reviews may be found on www.healthyeatingadvisor.com, amazon.com, dyingtolookgood.com, or at www.kiss4healthpublishing.com.